Lymphoproliferative Disorders:
Clinical, Immunologic and Morphological Correlation

Robert J. Lukes, M.D.
Professor of Pathology,
USC School of Medicine

and

John R. Craig, M.D., Ph.D.
Assistant Professor of Pathology,
USC School of Medicine

Published by

Symposia Specialists
Inc.
MEDICAL BOOKS

Distributed by

®

**YEAR BOOK
MEDICAL PUBLISHERS**
CHICAGO • LONDON

Symposia Specialists, Inc.
1470 N.E. 129th Street
Miami, FL 33161

Distributed by
Year Book Medical Publishers
35 E. Wacker Drive
Chicago, IL 60601

Library of Congress Catalog Number 79-88541
International Standard Book Number 0-8151-5646-4

Printed in the United States of America

Contents

III. T CELL LESIONS

IV. HISTIOCYTIC LESIONS

V. ABNORMAL IMMUNE REACTIONS: IMITATORS OF HODGKIN'S DISEASE

VI. HODGKIN'S DISEASE

Preface

The 62nd Semi-Annual Slide Seminar of the California Tumor Tissue Registry was presented by Professor Robert J. Lukes, M.D., on behalf of the California Tumor Tissue Registry which is a nonprofit voluntary professional organization that provides educational programs of special interest to pathologists. The semi-annual seminars usually include 25 case presentations with histologic slides and protocol (radiographs, if appropriate) mailed in advance to participants. Subsequently, an addendum is prepared and includes review of the individual subjects. Professor Robert J. Lukes, M.D., collected these 26 cases from his consultation files, the routine patient material at LAC-USC Medical Center and from the consultation files of the California Tumor Tissue Registry. Because of the prominent changes currently noted in hematopathology (stimulated in large part by Professor Lukes) it was desired to provide an updated proceedings for wider circulation than usual. Therefore, this volume has been published.

This volume includes information collated and provided by a group of investigators with specialized interest that allows more thorough individual case study than was possible several years ago. We wish to express appreciation to these many people who include John Parker, M.D., A. Delbert Cramer, M.D., William H. Sheehan, M.D., Barbara Tindle, M.D., Richard Neiman, M.D., Barbara K. Schneider, M.D., Clive Taylor, M.B. BChir, DPhil, Paul Pattengale, M.D., Thomas Lincoln, M.D., and many technologists who provided expertise in the functional studies of lymphocytes, immunoperoxidase staining technique and electron microscopy. The clinical evaluation was performed by a team including Don Feinstein, M.D., Alexandra Levine, M.D., Peter Rosen, M.D., and James Bonorris, M.D. Omission of certain key personnel in the above list is purely accidental.

This publication was prepared by review of the transcribed conference tape and subsequent review of each case with follow-up information. John R. Craig, M.D., Ph.D., Registrar of the California Tumor Tissue Registry, met with Professor Lukes two to three days a week for many months to discuss and outline various chapters and to review recent literature. During the time since the original presentation, follow-up of several cases has been useful in clarifying the condition and supporting the original interpretation. Many publications (over 50) by the USC Hematopathology group have appeared which support the original concepts presented. Although more documentation of each topic was originally desired, such as clinical staging data and treatment response of each condition, it seems prudent to present the pathologic information in these several cases and the more complete data obtained since that has been collated and evaluated. Professor Lukes has provided the interpretive hematopathologic expertise and Dr. Craig has assisted in the data organization, photography, literature review and revision of the manuscript. Each participant in the conference will receive this volume as part of the conference registration. Each case was accessioned into the files of the California Tumor Tissue Registry and is given an accession number (indicated by ACC).

W. K. Bullock, M.D.
Executive Director

Introduction

Modern concepts of normal immunologic function have challenged traditional histologic classification of the lymphoproliferative disorders. Furthermore the diagnosis and treatment of patients depend upon exact and precise histopathologic diagnosis. Therefore, a review of lymphoproliferative disorders and their classification with emphasis on histologic interpretation is valuable for the practicing hematopathologist, general pathologist, hematologist, oncologist and other physicians treating patients with these diseases. We have collected 26 representative cases to illustrate a variety of lymphoproliferative disorders covering the spectrum of multiple types of malignant lymphomas, immunoblastic sarcomas, T lymphocytic lesions, histiocytic lesions, abnormal reactions which mimic Hodgkin's disease and various subtypes of Hodgkin's disease. For each case the clinical features, gross and microscopic descriptions, histologic differential diagnosis, staging results and clinical correlation are presented with brief literature review.

Malignant lymphoma of B lymphocyte origin is represented by six examples involving lymph node and extranodal sites including lung, terminal ileum and thyroid. For historical interest, the bursa of Fabricius is described and illustrated. Reactive lymphoid hyperplasia in lymph node can be a challenging problem for the histopathologist and one example is discussed. In addition, an example of orbital granulocytic sarcoma submitted as Burkitt lymphoma is illustrated and the histological differential diagnosis is described.

Immunoblastic sarcoma, a recently described malignant disorder of transformed lymphocytes, is represented by five examples including one arising in the brain. The clinical and pathologic features of 33 patients are summarized.

T lymphocytes have been recognized as producing distinctive clinical pathologic syndromes and two such examples are described: the convoluted lymphocytic lymphoma-leukemia (T cell) arising in the mediastinum and mycosis fungoides involving skin and axillary lymph node.

The chapter on histiocytic lesions includes malignant histiocytosis, a rare but histologically distinctive condition, a true histiocytic malignant lymphoma and hairy cell leukemia involving the spleen (although the histiocytic origin of this condition is not certain).

The histopathologist recognizes several conditions that mimic Hodgkin's disease and are problems of histologic interpretation. Therefore, three examples of imitators of Hodgkin's disease are presented and include an exuberant immune reaction in lymph node, immunoblastic lymphadenopathy and a metastatic squamous carcinoma. A table of histologic criteria indicates the appropriate diagnostic clues and pitfalls for the histopathologist attempting to classify these cases.

Hodgkin's disease has a wide variety of histologic and clinical presentation and four examples cover several major histologic and clinical manifestations of this disease.

I
Malignant Lymphoma

Introduction

The classification of malignant lymphoma has traditionally been based upon histopathologic observation and correlation with clinical behavior. Although many refinements occurred over the decades, none of the previous classifications were based upon the normal function of the lymphocyte. With the recent understanding of normal lymphocyte function and stages of lymphocyte transformation, it became important to reexamine the classification of malignant lymphoma. Beginning with the fortuitous discovery by Glick of the function of the bursa of Fabricius as outlined in case 25, it subsequently became possible to classify circulating lymphocytes based on their function as thymus-derived or bursal-derived lymphocytes. These lymphocytes are related by function and the T derived lymphocytes are involved with cell-mediated immunity whereas the B derived lymphocytes are required for antibody formation. This classification scheme based on function was applied to the classification of malignant lymphoma. Furthermore, it was realized that malignant lymphomas were tumors of lymphocytes, but it was proposed that the neoplastic process was related to the lymphocyte transformation process. It was proposed that malignant lymphomas were aberrant forms of lymphocyte transformation and were a result of a block in the normal progression of transformation or the result of an inappropriate overabundant transformation process. To further examine these two proposals, namely (a) that lymphocytes could be related to the functional status (T or B cell) and (b) that malignant lymphoma was a result of aberrant lymphocyte transformation, a large-scale review and prospective study of lymphomatous disorders was undertaken. Several portions of these investigations have already been published [1-3]. In the recent review of 425 cases of malignant lymphoma, the functional studies allowed classification as outlined in Table 1.

Table 1. Distribution of Cases of Malignant Lymphomas by
Major Cytologic Group [1]

	No. of Cases	Percent
B cell	290	68.2
T cell	79	18.7
U cell (undefined)	55	12.9
Histiocytes	1	0.2
Total	425	100.0

Further refinement of this functional classification by addition of histologic criteria allows a number of subtypes as noted in Table 2.

These histologic criteria are based on cytologic criteria recognized from studies of lymphocyte transformation. Thus, the various steps of lymphocyte transformation may be represented by specific categories of the follicular center cell lymphomas. In review of these cases, it is important to

Table 2. Distribution of Cases of Malignant Lymphomas by
Cytologic Types of Lukes and Collins [1]

	No. of Cases	Percent
B cell		
Small lymphocyte (B)	39	9.2
Plasmacytoid lymphocyte	29	6.8
Follicular center cell (FCC)	(193)	(45.4)
Small cleaved	119	28.0
Large cleaved	21	4.9
Small noncleaved	29	6.8
Large noncleaved	24	5.7
Immunoblastic sarcoma (B)	15	3.5
Hairy cell leukemia	14	3.3
T cell		
Small lymphocyte (T)	10	2.4
Convoluted lymphocyte	41	9.7
Cerebriform lymphocyte (Sezary-Mycosis fungoides)	9	2.1
Immunoblastic sarcoma (T)	15	3.5
Lymphoepithelioid cell	4	1.0
Histiocytes	1	0.2
U Cell	55	12.9
Total	425	100.0

indicate that whereas more than 3,500 functional studies have been completed in our laboratory, refinements in the technique have occurred at times that have allowed more accurate results. For example, some cases present in a polyclonal manner and yet refinement in the technique with overnight incubation has revealed that some immunoglobulin was adherent and that monoclonal marking was the true marking of the cell. Thus, with experience, refinement in the functional technique has improved and allowed more accurate correlation and histologic interpretation. Furthermore, the cytologic criteria seemed to us to be of greatest prognostic importance rather than the observation of the follicular or diffuse nature of the neoplasm.

The classification scheme based on function and histologic criteria is reproducible and clinical applications to large groups of specific types are now in progress. The prognostic value of this scheme is under study in several centers.

Clinical Staging

The critical moment for clinical staging in patients with this disorder is at the time of primary surgery. Unfortunately, this factor may not be appreciated at the time of surgery. The pathologist may play an active role at the time of surgery and can make an important contribution by encouraging detailed examination of mesenteric nodes, search of the abdomen and completion of the staging. The abdomen should be searched for involvement in the liver, spleen, periaortic nodes and a wedge biopsy of the posterior iliac crest marrow obtained. It is recommended that lymph nodes be obtained from the left periaortic region, celiac axis and the splenic hilar region. Two needle biopsies of the liver and a wedge biopsy of the liver are generally obtained. Splenectomy in childhood has more recently raised an issue because of the increased frequency of pneumococcal septicemia developing in a small number of children. Therefore, splenectomy is not recommended in children, whereas in an adult because this septicemia has been rare, splenectomy is generally not as hazardous.

If lymphomatous nodules are discernible visually in the liver, then splenectomy is not required for staging. Because the small noncleaved FCC type involves the spleen in an irregular and nodular fashion, it commonly may be grossly evident in the spleen. Therefore, even though the spleen is not removed in a child, the spleen should be carefully examined for involvement. The pathologist, aware of the conditions for staging in both Hodgkin's disease and non-Hodgkin's lymphomas in various situations, can contribute importantly to patient care at the time of surgery. In addition, the pathologist's presence in the operating room will permit him to achieve the essential ideal fixation and preparation of tissue imprints to characterize the cytologic details properly.

Additional Studies

The laboratory techniques for the functional studies have been described by Lukes et al [3]. The chart in the tables of the various sections indicates the functional studies by abbreviation. These abbreviations are as follows:

E	T (E Rosette)
EA	Histiocyte/Monocyte
EAC	B (Complement Receptor)
PV	*Polyvalent Heavy Chain
M	*Heavy Chain M
G	*Heavy Chain G
A	*Heavy Chain A
D	*Heavy Chain D
κ	*Light Chain Kappa
λ	*Light Chain Lambda

As previously mentioned, a word of caution is important in interpreting the functional studies. We have found several examples of polyclonal markings which upon restudy have indicated monoclonal marking, and the revised results were more in keeping with the cytologic criteria and histopathologic interpretation. We currently believe that the histopathologic criteria are essential in the appropriate classification and that the failure to find monoclonal marking does not disprove the presence of lymphoma. As review of the several cases in this conference will illustrate, some

---

*SIg = Surface immunoglobulin by immunofluorescence.

recognized entities of lymphoreticular disorders have consistently marked in a polyclonal fashion and appropriate discussion is provided for these cases. In the past year use of prior incubation for at least 45 minutes and $F(ab')_2$ antisera reagents for SIg have greatly reduced the problem of polyclonicity.

References

1. Lukes, R.J., Parker, J.W. et al: Immunologic approach to non-Hodgkin's lymphomas and related disorders. Analysis of the results of multiparameter studies of 425 cases. Semin. Hematol. 5:322-351, 1978.
2. Lukes, R.J. and Collins, R.D.: Immunologic characterization of human malignant lymphomas. Cancer 34:1488-1503, 1974.
3. Lukes, R.J., Taylor, C.R. et al: A morphologic and immunologic surface marker study of 299 cases of non-Hodgkin lymphomas and related leukemias. Am. J. Pathol. 90:461-486, 1978.

Bibliography

Lukes, R.J. and Peckham, N.T.: Non-Hodgkin's lymphoma: A retrospective analysis of major prognostic factors including histopathology. (Submitted for publication.)
Strauchen, J., Young, R.C. and DeVita, V.T.: Clinical relevance of the histopath subclassification of diffuse histiocytic lymphoma. N. Engl. J. Med. (In press.)

Bursa of Fabricius, Chicken

Clinical History

This specimen is a bursa of Fabricius obtained from a chicken from a local animal processing plant.

Microscopic Findings

A saclike structure is outlined by a connective tissue capsule at the periphery and multiple villous projections containing prominent lymphoid follicles. The villi are covered by tall columnar epithelial cells with nuclei in the basal area. The epithelial layer is uniform and forms many invaginations within the underlying submucosal tissue. In the submucosal tissue are exuberant lymphoid follicles of fairly uniform size which are separated by very thin fibrous septae. These follicles contain a wide range of cell nuclei typical of small to large lymphocytes. Some of the larger nuclei contain prominent nucleoli that are centrally located and others are peripherally located adjacent to the nuclear rim. Many nuclei have prominent nuclear cleaves and the amount of cytoplasm is variable. A few areas between the follicles reveal small vessels containing nucleated red blood cells typical of avian circulating red blood cells.

Discussion

Fabricius studied the saclike gland in the chicken 300 years ago at Padua. Of interest is that his studies apparently led Harvey, another student at Padua, to his concept of the circulation. The bursa, later named after Fabricius, is a round or pear-shaped diverticulum on the dorsal aspect of the avian cloaca [1]. Inside the sac are many villous structures containing prominent lymphoid follicles. The villi are covered with columnar epithelial cells and this forms a structure that resembles the thymus.

The function of the bursa has been disputed for centuries and was attributed to many different functions including semen reservoir, urinary bladder, egg reservoir, seminal vesicle, prostate, anal gland, Cowper's gland and cecum. Because the bursa involution coincides with chicken sexual maturity, a primary role in sexual maturity was suggested. Furthermore, it was suggested that the bursa suppressed testicular growth and when the bursa involuted, the testes were allowed to mature. Others proposed that the gland was involved in nutrition and absorption from the GI tract, while there were those who suggested a role in hematopoiesis. The normal growth of the bursa has been well studied and varies in different types of birds. The most rapid growth occurs in the young bird prior to 4 weeks of age and regression in weight occurs after it has attained maximum size which is approximately 11 to 13 weeks [2].

The association of antibody production with the presence of the bursa was a monumental but accidental discovery of Glick reported in 1956 [3]. He was searching for a source of chicken blood with a high titer of Salmonella typhimurium antibody for use in other experiments. Therefore, he injected inactivated cultures into chickens. By chance a surplus of female chickens that had been bursectomized previously at 12 days of age was available for test injection. Six birds previously bursectomized died after the injection and three survivors produced no antibodies. The nonbursectomized females were unaffected and had normal titers of the Salmonella antibody. Therefore, he systematically studied this relationship of bursectomy to failure to produce Salmonella antibody in these young chickens.

Subsequent studies have indicated that cortisol and androgenic hormones cause involution of the bursa. Thus, the role of the bursa in sexual maturity is quite the reverse than was expected. In fact, hormonal manipulation is used to produce a chemical bursectomy which is valuable in research studies of the bursa.

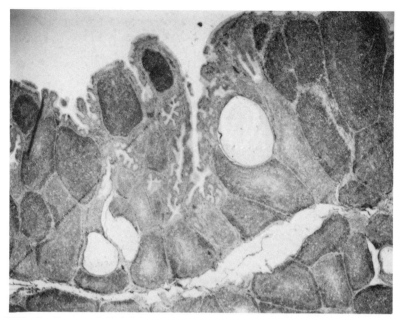

FIG. 1. Bursa of Fabricius is composed of lymphoid follicles of fairly uniform shape and a villous lining of tall columnar epithelial cells (H & E 12.5×).

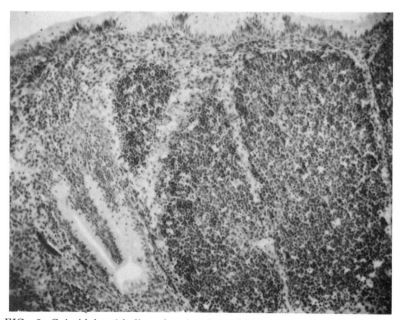

FIG. 2. Cuboidal epithelium has basal nuclei and many enfoldings producing glandular clefts adjacent to lymphoid follicles (H & E 50×).

References

1. Glick, B.: The bursa of Fabricius and development of immunologic competence. *In* Good, R.A. and Gabrielson, A.E. (eds.): The Thymus in Immunobiology. Harper & Row, New York, 1964, Chap. 19.
2. Glick, B.: Normal growth of the bursa of Fabricius in chickens. Poult. Sci. 35:843-851, 1956.
3. Glick, B., Chang, T.S. and Jaap, R.G.: Research notes. The bursa of Fabricius and antibody production. Poult. Sci. 35:224-225, 1956.

Reactive Hyperplasia, Follicular and Perisinusoidal Cell, Cervical Lymph Node

Clinical History

This 7-year-old Mexican-American female had an enlarged left neck mass for several months. She was scheduled for elective resection of probable branchial cleft cyst. The patient previously had a hernia repair in 1971, tonsillectomy and adenoidectomy in 1974 and viral hepatitis in February of 1976. She also was mentally retarded and had chronic left otitis media. Physical examination demonstrated bilaterally scarred ear drums and a 3 × 2 cm cystic mass in the superior third of the left sternocleidal mastoid muscle. The mass was mobile and nontender. Laboratory studies showed a hemoglobin of 12.4 gm% and a WBC of 7200 cells/mm^3. Bilateral myringotomies and an excision of the left neck mass were performed.

Gross Pathology

The neck mass specimen was 3 × 2 × 2 cm soft oval tan tissue.

Microscopic Findings

This lymph node exhibits two striking features, prominent follicular hyperplasia, and zones of mononuclear cells situated beneath the capsule and as interconnecting foci in the interfollicular tissue. The follicular structures are greatly enlarged, often oval or elongated, and even dumbbell shaped, but in general they vary prominently in size. The most impressive feature is the presence of starry-sky phagocytes that contain prominent nuclear debris. Often the lymphocytic mantles around the follicles are not prominent and at times the follicles are devoid of this zone of lymphocytes. On closer examination of the follicular centers, there is a mixed composition with a prominent component of large mononuclear cells for which we have given the term, the noncleaved follicular center cells (NC FCC). In addition, there are small cells with scanty cytoplasm and irregular nuclear configuration, some of which have deep nuclear cleavage planes, and these have been designated the cleaved follicular center cell (FCC). In general, these two types of cells are arranged in an irregular mixture, though in areas the large noncleaved cells are arranged at one margin, and a few even appear to be separating into the adjacent zone of lymphocytes. The large noncleaved cells have finely dispersed chromatin and usually several small to intermediate size irregular nucleoli often situated on the nuclear membrane.

On close inspection a moderate amount of lightly basophilic cytoplasm is present that is strikingly pyroninophilic. The noncleaved cells exhibit a wide range in size from approximately 2 to 5 lymphocyte nuclear diameters. The phagocytes have abundant pale acidophilic cytoplasm with ill-defined cellular borders and prominent phagocytic nuclear debris of varying size and configuration. These nuclei of phagocytes are usually large, oval in configuration with a medium size centrally situated nucleolus. The large noncleaved FCC cells have nuclei that are larger than the histiocyte nucleus. In the interfollicular tissue there are foci of cytoplasmic cohesive mononuclear cells with rather small to intermediate size irregular nuclei. These foci are similar to the zones of mononuclear cells beneath the capsule and in general follow the sinusoidal distribution. In a few areas an adjacent or several sinusoidal lumens can be seen. These sinusoids contain similar scattered detached cytoplasmic mononuclear cells. We have designated these cells "perisinusoidal" cells on the basis of their association with lymph node sinuses and the infrequency of demonstrating the cells within the sinusoid lumen. The cellular borders are cohesive and on close inspection an interlocking cellular border at times can be discerned.

Special Studies

Immunoperoxidase studies for cytoplasmic immunoglobulin reveal the large noncleaved FCC contain either kappa or lambda light chains and do not appear monoclonal. Acid phosphatase stains on frozen section of the fresh tissue were done. Perisinusoidal cells reveal strong positivity in the largest cells and no staining for the majority. Using tartrate blocking several of the cells retain their positivity in slight degree. Immunologic surface marking studies were performed on suspensions of fresh cells prepared from this lymph node. The results demonstrate typical features that we have found in a large number of reactive lymph nodes. There were 57% E rosettes for T cells, and polyclonal surface marking of a small proportion of the cells for B cells.

Histologic Differential Diagnosis

The differential diagnosis is concerned with the two distinctive components. The follicular proliferation of this type in the past gave rise to the problem of so-called Brill-Symmers disease and required differentiation of giant follicular hyperplasia and follicular lymphoma. With the passage of time and acquisition of experience, and the contribution of Dr. Henry Rappaport, we believe the histological differential diagnosis has become easier. We have come to appreciate that variability in size and configuration of the follicles are usually associated with benign reactive hyperplasia. The second important feature is the presence of phagocytosis which almost always is associated with reactive follicles. Only on rare occasions are reactive phagocytes of so-called starry-sky type found in lymphomatous follicles (nodular lymphomas). The final feature of clinical importance is the age of the patients. Lymphomas with a follicular or non-follicular pattern rarely occur under the age of 30, and follicular lymphoma is almost nonexistent under the age of 20.

The second component, the perisinusoidal proliferation, is striking because of the abundance noted in this case and presents considerable difficulty for the pathologist unfamiliar with this cellular proliferation. Its common location beneath the capsule raises the question of a metastatic neoplasm of unusual type. The differentiation is based upon the long zones of these cells perfectly following sinusoids, composed of cohesive cells with pale cytoplasm, ill-defined cellular borders and the rarity of sinusoidal lumen. In addition, the nuclei are rather small and fairly uniform in configuration and lack anaplastic features. In general, they do not resemble any common metastatic epithelial tumor. Most commonly, the presence of these cells would raise the question of a drainage reaction and an inflammatory response.

Some reactions produce necrotizing granulomata and these are (1) tularemia; (2) cat-scratch fever; (3) Yersinia intercolitica; and (4) lymphogranuloma venereum. These lesions are essentially indistinguishable from each other and are differentiated by other immunologic techniques. Finally, the perisinusoidal cells in our experience are most commonly noted in toxoplasmosis with follicular hyperplasia and a typical distribution of the histiocytes in relationship to follicular center cells. The typical histiocytes of toxoplasmosis are lacking in this case.

Clinical Correlation and Follow-up

Prominent follicular hyperplasia has been observed in a wide variety of situations often without any suggestion to indicate a specific etiology. In association with perisinusoidal cells, it has been most commonly found with toxoplasmosis, but then accompanied by clusters of histiocytes in the lymphocytic mantle and in interfollicular locations. We cannot recall a similar case in which these two components, the dramatic follicular hyperplasia and striking degree of perisinusoidal cells, have been observed together. Therefore, it is impossible to provide specific clinical correlations because of the uniqueness of this case. Both features, however, from our general experience are indicative of an immunologic response of benign type and in themselves are not specific. The perisinusoidal reaction in addition to toxoplasmosis appears to be a frequent component in minor degrees in reactive processes. It also occurs in cat-scratch fever, tularemia, Yersinia intercolitica and lymphogranuloma venereum in association with necrotizing granulomas apparently as part of the regional drainage reaction response. In general, it appears that this cellular proliferation is not etiologically specific, though it may represent a significant cellular component in immunologic reaction, the precise nature of which we are presently not aware.

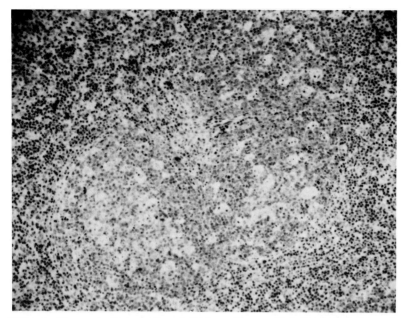

FIG. 1. Hyperplastic reactive follicle with an ill-defined lymphocytic mantle. Starry-sky pattern of phagocytes is prominent (H & E 50×).

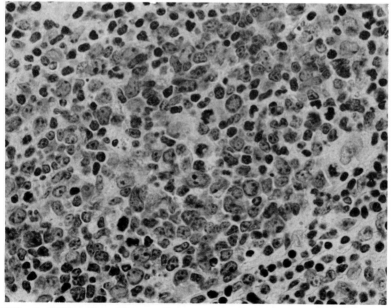

FIG. 2. FCC cells with prominent component of noncleaved cells and numerous mitoses. Smaller irregular component represents the small cleaved FCC component (H & E 50×).

Malignant Lymphoma, Small Cleaved and Large Noncleaved Follicular Center Cell, Follicular and Diffuse, Inguinal Lymph Node

Clinical History

This 70-year-old female was noted to have left inguinal lymphadenopathy on routine physical examination. There was no evidence of injury or inflammation in the area or in the leg. Subsequent physical examination revealed possible enlargement of the inguinal lymph nodes which were smooth, movable and nontender. An excisional biopsy of the right inguinal nodes was performed.

Gross Pathology

A cordlike mass of yellow lobulated fatty tissue measuring up to 10.0 × 2.5 × 2.0 cm was removed. On one pole of the mass was a large encapsulated gray-tan oval 4.5 × 2.5 × 2.2 cm nodule. The cut surface was homogenous, fleshy, nonbulging tissue with focal areas of hemorrhage. Multiple other small gray-tan nodes measuring up to 2.3 cm in greatest dimension were found in the remaining fatty tissue.

Microscopic Findings

This lymph node specimen was selected for the conference because it exhibited a number of features of follicular center cell (FCC) lymphoma with areas that are distinctly follicular (nodular) in distribution and other areas that are diffuse. The cytologic type also varies from small cleaved to large noncleaved

FCC type. Thus, in one specimen most of the morphologic expressions of the FCC lymphomas can be observed.

At one end of the lymph node, follicular structures with ill-defined margins and broad lymphocytic mantles can be noted. In one area (A), the follicles are composed somewhat of a mixture of large noncleaved cells with prominent cytoplasm. Similar cells are found in the interfollicular tissue in varying numbers. In the diffuse areas of the node (B), the proliferation is predominately small cleaved FCC with a range of cell size. This cellular infiltration extends broadly through the capsule. In the third area (C), the well-defined follicular structures are composed predominately of large cytoplasmic cells, and in areas this proliferation extends into the interfollicular tissue where the margins are ill-defined. A careful examination of the three areas and the cytologic types within reveals the size variation of the cleaved FCC and the remarkable degree of irregularity and nuclear subdivisions that may be seen within the cleaved FCC. Thus, this small proliferation ranges widely in size from that of a small lymphocyte to a large lymphocyte with abundant cytoplasm although the smaller component predominates.

The noncleaved FCC also range in size in the specimen and, for the most part, are oval or round in configuration. Their cytoplasm is generally prominent; their cellular borders are frequently well demarcated. Typically, this proliferation will be strikingly pyroninophilic.

Special Studies

The lymph node cells were collected for our multiparameter studies. Over 60% of the cells had surface immunoglobulin in a monoclonal fashion as IgM kappa. The remaining cells marked with E rosettes as T cells. These findings support the B cell nature of this lymphoma and are typical of the FCC lymphomas.

	E	EAC	EA	PV	M	G	A	D	κ	λ
Lymph node	35	ND		63	62	0	0	8	53	14

Histologic Differential Diagnosis

There are two major considerations in the differential diagnosis: (1) benign reactive hyperplasia and (2) malignant lymphoma. In addition, another problem exists relative to the precise categorization within the follicular center cell lymphoma. The follicular center cell lymphomas with the four cytologic components in the natural evolution of the malignant process range from the low turnover rate, small cleaved FCC type, to the large noncleaved FCC. As the process evolves, we can categorize the first expression under the single general category of the FCC group. In the past, a change in terminology was always necessary (such as the poorly differentiated lymphocytic type, nodular to the histiocytic type). The differentiation between reactive follicular hyperplasia and lymphomas with a follicular pattern has been the subject of debate for decades. The recent establishment of lymphomas with a nodular pattern as lymphomatous follicles composed of follicular center cells demonstrates the reason why the differentiation, at times, may be difficult [1, 2]. From our experience, the histologic diagnosis of a lymphoma of follicular center cell type is based upon the cellular composition of the follicles and cytologic criteria rather than on the general features of follicle size and configuration, although the latter provide helpful guidelines. Identification of lymphoma cells in the interfollicular tissue is one of the most helpful features in the recognition of these lymphomas. The most reliable histologic features are noted in Table 1.

A predominance of a single cell type usually occurs and in the small cleaved FCC is over 90% and the large noncleaved FCC is over 70% homogenous [3]. The FCC lymphomas essentially *are always* mixtures of cleaved and noncleaved cells, but essentially one or the other cell predominates. In the small cleaved FCC lymphoma, usually the large noncleaved occurs in low percentage (1% to 5% or 10% and rarely approaches 20%). The size and configuration of the follicles in this case fit with the FCC type of lymphoma. The small cleaved FCC are ill-defined and are composed of blue staining cells with scanty

Table 1. Features Favoring Lymphoma Rather Than Reactive Process

1. Cytologic criteria — predominant cell type

2. Absence of phagocytosis

3. Extension of proliferation into interfollicular area

4. Extension of proliferation through capsule

cytoplasm; the infiltrate extends through the interfollicular tissue and capsule. With an increase in the number of large noncleaved cells or large cleaved cells, more cytoplasm is apparent; the follicular centers appear acidophilic and a lymphocytic mantle becomes apparent. With these types of lymphomatous structures the resemblance to reactive follicles is more apparent and differentiation is more difficult. In these situations estimation of the number of large noncleaved cells is very helpful, but final determination and solution of the problem may be readily achieved by examination of the interfollicular tissue, the capsule and the finding of small or large cleaved FCC types. The presence of phagocytes favors a reactive process and "starry-sky phagocytes" are rare in lymphomatous follicles and a reliable indicator of caution against lymphoma. Certain features of reactive follicles are helpful. Reactive follicles are commonly larger, more irregular in configuration and have more sharply demarcated reaction centers. The cellular composition is usually dramatically mixed. In exuberant reactive follicles, large noncleaved cells may be prominent but are intermixed typically with starry-sky phagocytes. Capsular infiltration in small foci, particularly about vessels, may be observed in a variety of reactive processes, but essentially never as broad areas of infiltration involving much of the capsule as seen in the FCC lymphomas. Thus, there are numerous features in this specimen that lead to a diagnosis of lymphoma.

Classification of this process with the FCC lymphomas is difficult, and we have chosen to emphasize that two prominent areas contain the small cleaved and the large noncleaved FCC. In the past, the findings of separate areas of involvement by different cytologic types of lymphomas usually were designated as a composite lymphoma and the two areas listed separately [4]. In this case, we are observing several different expressions of the follicular center cell lymphoma, and it does not in a sense fulfill the criteria for a composite lymphoma. Of major concern in classifying the follicular center cell lymphomas is the evolution to the high turnover rate type, the small or large noncleaved FCC, since the prognosis relates directly to their presence. Thus, if a portion of the node is composed entirely by the noncleaved FCC type, it deserves emphasis even though the majority of the node is composed of either the small or large cleaved type, since the prognosis appears to be dependent upon the most aggressive component which is the noncleaved FCC.

The findings in these nodes do not raise the question of any other malignancy, such as a metastatic neoplasm.

Clinical Staging

No special procedures were done for staging. A bone marrow examination did not reveal any evidence of lymphoma.

Clinical Correlation and Follow-up

The follicular center cell lymphomas most commonly present as asymptomatic peripheral lymphadenopathy that often seems to be limited to a single region, but on careful staging the process is generalized. As frequently encountered, dissemination of this disease in our experience relates to the presence of the small cleaved FCC type which is commonly found in the majority of the cases. This cell type apparently circulates widely and it involves the bone marrow to such a degree that probably over 70% of the cases have bone marrow involvement if abundant marrow is obtained for examination. If the process is essentially of the small cleaved cell type, it is of low aggressiveness despite wide distribution. If a large noncleaved cell component is prominent or dominates a portion of the node, the process appears to be changing in the aggressiveness. The presence of noncleaved FCC is commonly associated with lymph node enlargement and it is often accompanied by the development of symptomatic disease and the rapid development of many lymph node masses. Furthermore, failure on previously effective chemotherapy regimens also may be encountered and a change in course is a demonstration of the need for sequential lymph node biopsies. Such patients often exhibit a predominant noncleaved FCC pattern. Thus, the prognosis in the FCC lymphoma depends upon whether the predominant cells are the slowly progressing small cleaved FCC type or the high turnover large noncleaved FCC. Furthermore, the process can change from the former to the latter. In the small cleaved FCC type with some degree of follicular pattern the median survival is approximately seven years, whereas it is less than one year with a large noncleaved FCC type. Thus, a patient who has progressed slowly for a number of years may abruptly change to the high turnover rate, and then the prognosis and expected median survival is that of the newly apparent large noncleaved FCC.

This patient was alive and well 18 months after diagnosis but lost to follow-up at 21 months.

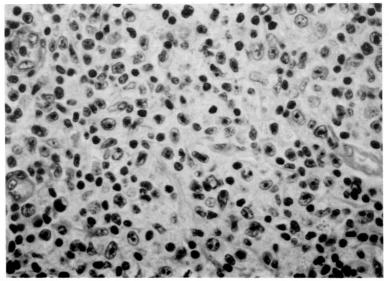

FIG. 1. This unusual pattern of nodal involvement exhibits both prominent follicular and interfollicular lymphomatous proliferation (H & E 12.5×).

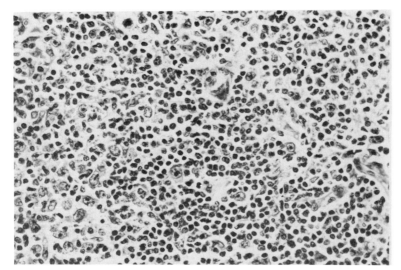

FIG. 2. Lymphomatous follicular centers are predominantly small cleaved cells with varying mixtures of large noncleaved FCC (H & E 125×).

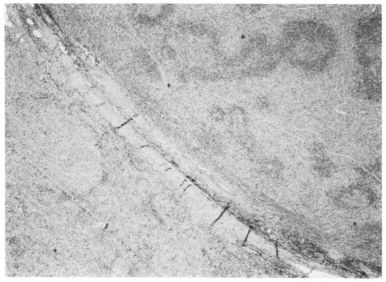

FIG. 3. Interfollicular tissue is composed of predominantly small cleaved cells, a small component of large noncleaved FCC and intercellular amorphous material (H & E 500×).

References

1. Jaffe, E.S., Shevach, E.M. and Frank, M.M.: Nodular lymphoma —
   Evidence for origin from follicular lymphocytes. N. Engl. J. Med.
   290:813-819, 1974.
2. Levine, G. and Dorfman, R.: Nodular lymphoma: An ultrastructural
   study of its relationship to germinal centers and a correlation of LM
   and EM. Cancer 35:148, 1975.
3. Glick, A.D., Leech, J.A., Waldron, J.A. et al: Ultrastructural and
   cytochemical studies. J. Natl. Cancer Inst. 54:23-36, 1975.
4. Kim, H., Hendrickson, M.R. and Dorfman, R.F.: Composite
   lymphoma. Cancer 40:959-976, 1977.

Malignant Lymphoma, Small Cleaved Follicular Center Cell, Diffuse, Axillary Lymph Node

Clinical History

This 80-year-old female noted a lump in the right arm for approximately six months. The arm mass was excised in October 1975 and the bone marrow and blood findings were normal. She was hospitalized in November 1975 for a biopsy and axillary node dissection. At the time of admission for the axillary node biopsy, physical examination showed a hard fixed mass overlying the healed incisional scar of the right arm just above the elbow and one large palpable lymph node in the right axilla. The peripheral blood findings, chest radiograph and liver-spleen scan were interpreted as normal.

Gross Pathology

A right axillary lymph node dissection yielded multiple lymph nodes ranging in size from 2.5 to 5.0 cm. The cut surface of each of the nodes was tan, glistening and homogenous.

Microscopic Findings

The axillary node on low magnification revealed a diffuse involvement with infiltration of the capsule and no discernible nodularity or follicles. The cellular proliferation is fairly uniform and composed of small lymphocytic-type cells. The nuclear configuration is irregular and cytoplasm is scanty or indistinct without cohesive cellular borders. Nuclear cleavage planes are found in a small proportion of the cells. The nuclear chromatin is compact and nucleoli essentially are absent. A variable number of somewhat larger cells with irregular nuclei and finer nuclear chromatin are scattered throughout the

27

diffuse proliferation. The methyl green pyronine stained sections show these scattered larger cells have pyroninophilic cytoplasm and finely dispersed nuclear chromatin often with several small nucleoli. Mitoses are rare. The original biopsy in the right arm revealed a similar cellular proliferation. In the Rappaport classification, the process could be considered either in the well-differentiated lymphocytic type, diffuse, if the observer felt the cells were small, or in the poorly differentiated lymphocytic type if he considered them sufficiently large.

Special Studies

Tissue was collected for immunologic surface marker and ultrastructural studies on this case. The majority of the cells marked as B cells with almost 80% of the cells having IgM heavy chain on their surface without IgG, IgA or IgD. However, both kappa and lambda chains were identified on the surface, forming an unusual or anomalous bitypic light chain pattern. We suspect this abnormality is probably due to a crossover and a nonspecific marking of one of the light chains. Only a small proportion of the cells (less than 10%) marked with E rosettes for T cells. A parallel study of the surface marker techniques on the peripheral blood lymphocytes demonstrated that over 60% of the cells marked with E rosettes for T cells and less than 10% with surface immunoglobulins for B cells without any evidence of monoclonality.

Peripheral	E	EAC	EA	PV	M	G	A	D	κ	λ
blood	63	ND	ND	8	2	3	0	0	4	1
Lymph node	8	0	0	87	74	0	0	0	71	77

Histologic Differential Diagnosis

The problem for the pathologist in evaluating such lesions primarily is concerned with differentiating cytologic types of lymphomas of the relatively small cell type. These categories include the small B lymphocyte, small T lymphocyte and the plasmacytoid lymphocyte types. At times, an extranodal pseudolymphomatous reaction may be difficult to classify. Differentiation of these types depends upon the availability of thin, well-stained histologic sections of no greater than 5 μ in thickness. This is important since lymphocytes in histologic sections measure approximately 4 μ and thicker sections produce overlapping and stratification of lymphocytes. Recognition of the small cleaved lymphocytic cell is dependent upon the finding of nuclear cleavage planes, compact chromatin and irregular nuclear configuration. In the small B lymphocytic lymphoma, the proliferation is a small round lymphocyte with scanty cytoplasm without plasmacytoid cells, whereas the small T lymphocyte is a somewhat irregular nucleus with "knuckle-like" protrusions usually on one surface. The number of cases with ideal histologic material we have been able to study is too limited to provide an ideal differential diagnostic criteria at this time. The plasmacytoid lymphocytic lymphoma is characterized by a range of cells from the small lymphocyte to a plasmacytoid cell with a lymphocyte type of ncleus with intermediate forms. The number of cells with plasmacytoid cytoplasm varies widely. Methyl green pyronine stains are commonly necessary to demonstrate the plasmacytoid cytoplasm. The finding of PAS positive intranuclear globules, the so-called Dutcher bodies, of IgM gammopathy is particularly useful in the plasmacytoid lymphocytic type of lymphoma. The most difficult differential diagnosis in extranodal tissues is the pseudolymphomatous reaction. These disorders may be diffuse and infiltrative without reactive follicles; and the differentiation between the small cleaved FCC type, diffuse and the pseudolymphoma is dependent upon the recognition of the cytologic type in the lymphoma and the mixture of cell types in the pseudolymphomatous reaction. Thus, when reactive follicular centers are present, the diagnosis of a pseudolymphoma is rather easy, but in their absence it is based upon mixture cells, including reactive plasma cells, histiocytes and a range of lymphocytes without nuclear cleavage planes.

Clinical Staging

No evidence to suggest malignant lymphoma outside of the axillary and deltoid region was demonstrated with conventional clinical staging techniques. Bone marrow evaluation failed to reveal any evidence of malignant lymphoma. Thus, the patient appeared to have disease limited to the axillary lymph node and deltoid mass and was regarded as clinical stage IE.

Clinical Correlation and Follow-up

This process even though diffuse is regarded as a low turn-over rate type of cellular proliferation that most commonly has distributed widely by the time of initial observation and most often has involvement of retroperitoneal lymph nodes, bone marrow and even spleen. In this case, it is possible that the bone marrow, despite a single adequate marrow sample, may have been involved in a minor degree that was difficult to detect. Bilateral iliac crest biopsies are often needed to detect small lesions. The patient was treated with regional radiation therapy to the right arm and axilla (10/76) and chemotherapy. Six months later recurrence in the submandibular area was detected. Chemotherapy was given (cytoxan, prednisone, vincristine). Eleven months after diagnosis she was readmitted with a hemoglobin of 8.5 gm% and given additional radiation and chemotherapy.

Malignant Lymphoma, Small Cleaved Follicular Center Cell, Diffuse, Lung

Clinical History

This 68-year-old black female complained of left shoulder and neck pain of six months duration. She denied any respiratory symptoms and did not smoke. Chest radiographs revealed a left hilar and parenchymal mass and she was admitted for further evaluation in October 1976. Physical examination indicated occasional ronchi and moist rales in the midleft lung field. Laboratory data included negative skin tests and negative sputum cytology. Bronchoscopy indicated an infiltrating lesion at the left lower lobe orifice with deformity of subsegmental bronchi. Biopsy and brushings were negative and mediastinoscopy of carinal and left mediastinal lymph nodes revealed no tumor. On October 26, 1976, a left pneumonectomy was performed.

Gross Pathology

The lung had a shiny, bluish-gray pleural surface, except in the lingula which was whitish-tan. Although the surgical margin of the bronchus was normal, sections of the distal bronchial tree revealed infiltration by tumor. The bronchial mucosa was yellowish-white, smooth and glistening. Eight parabronchial lymph nodes, the largest measuring up to 1.1 cm in diameter, were dark black, soft and homogenous. The lingular lobe was firm and whitish-tan on cut section, and the pulmonary arteries contained a reddish-black thrombus near the surgical margin extending into the left upper lobe.

Microscopic Findings

There is an infiltrative mass with only a few discernible bronchioles interspersed, and a few sections show alveoli with

31

septa infiltrated by tumor. On closer inspection, there are small and irregular, ill-defined follicular centers composed of a mixture of small and large noncleaved FCC types with the latter predominating. Phagocytes usually are not present, but a few reactive appearing plasma cells are found. Between these follicles and the small, compressed bronchioles, the cellular proliferation is predominately lymphocytic and abnormal by cytologic criteria. The lymphocytes are small, irregular, and a small component of these cells have nuclear cleavage planes. The nuclear chromatin is compact and basophilic; nucleoli are inapparent. The cytoplasm is somewhat prominent, pale staining and cells in areas appear to have a cohesive character with interlocking cellular borders. The latter feature is most unusual for a benign lymphocytic proliferation. Intermixed in variable proportions are small numbers of benign appearing immunoblasts. Irregularly distributed throughout the specimen is a component of perivascular hyalinized connective tissue that in a few areas is aggregated and forms dense foci. The bronchiolar epithelium reveals a range of cell size with a predominance in areas of a medium-sized cytoplasmic cohesive cell with an oval to irregular nucleus and interspersed large cells with finely dispersed chromatin and small nucleoli. A comparison of the medium-sized cell component with the lymphoma cells demonstrates a sufficient similarity that difficulty may be encountered if these cytologic details are not well portrayed, particularly on improperly fixed material.

Special Studies

In the ultrastructural studies the nuclear cleavage planes are more readily demonstrated and the lymphocytes have a moderate amount of cytoplasm and interlocking cellular borders as suspected in the histologic sections. Cell suspensions were collected for immunologic surface marker studies. Fourteen percent of the cells marked for T cells with E rosettes. Only a small proportion of cells marked in the EAC rosette studies, a finding that is commonly elevated when the cellular proliferation exhibits a prominent follicular pattern. The immunoperoxidase stain shows the tumor cells are negative. The finding of both kappa and lambda typing on functional studies indicates either absorption or polyclonal cells are present. Admittedly, the special studies do not support a monoclonal cell proliferation, but repeat testing is requested since some cases have been found to have technical artifact [1]. Thus, the morphological criteria are considered most reliable in this case.

	E	EAC	EA	PV	M	G	A	D	κ	λ
Lung Mass	14	4	2	83	78	50	0	31	83	52

Histologic Differential Diagnosis

The diagnostic problem for the pathologist in this case involves differentiation of a pseudolymphomatous reaction from malignant lymphoma. In the clinical setting presented by this case, the process most commonly will prove to be a pseudolymphoma, but this remarkable case challenges our morphologic criteria for the differentiation. Thus, in the lung almost all lymphoid masses of lymphocytic type with reactive follicles are pseudolymphoma, but an exceptional case may prove to be lymphomatous as exemplified by this case [2]. The criteria for diagnosing a pseudolymphoma are (1) the proliferation is primarily mixed in character, though predominantly lymphocytic, (2) reactive follicles are present, though at times few in number, and (3) plasma cells of reactive type and histiocytes with acidophilic cytoplasm usually with intermixed immunoblasts are present. In this process the lymphocytes are small, have round nuclei with compact chromatin, scanty or indistinct cytoplasm and noncohesive cellular borders. In the present case, the lymphocytes are abnormal with irregular nuclear configuration, nuclear cleavage planes, prominent cytoplasm and cohesive cellular borders. Admittedly, a few residual reactive follicles are present as are an occasional plasma cell and scattered immunoblasts.

Clinical Staging

The patient was thoroughly evaluated by our clinical staging approach, and no evidence of lymphoma could be detected by lymphangiography, scanning procedures or bone marrow examination.

Clinical Correlation and Follow-up

The presentation of a lymphoid mass in the lung without preceding evidence of a lymphoma elsewhere clinically fits well with a pseudolymphoma of the lung. This case presents an extraordinary situation in which the clinical presentation and several morphologic features fit well with a pseudolymphoma, but the cytologic details and ultrastructural studies provide evidence of a lymphomatous process. The situation in this case, therefore, raises three possibilities: (1) that a malignant lymphoma may develop as a primary lymphoma in the lung and have associated reactive follicles; (2) that a lymphoma may develop subsequent to pseudolymphomatous reaction; and (3) that a lymphoma may involve the lung secondarily in a patient who has a malignant lymphoma in lymph nodes elsewhere that are undetected by currently available techniques.

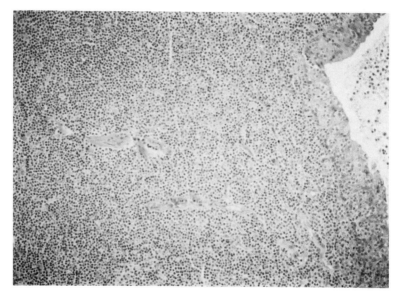

FIG. 1. There is diffuse proliferation of small lymphocytes throughout the lung mass with occasional space lined by proliferative epithelium. A few thick-walled small vessels are present (H & E 50×).

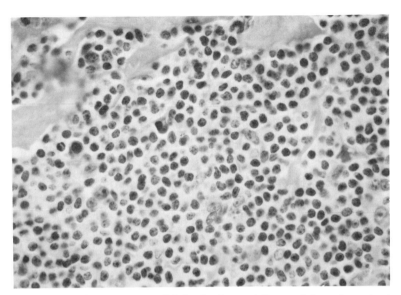

FIG. 2. Lymphocytes vary slightly in size and the nuclei are irregular in configuration with a small number having deep nuclear cleavage planes (H & E 500×).

References

1. Lukes, R.J., Taylor, C.R., Parker, J.W. et al: A morphologic and immunologic surface marker study of 299 cases of non-Hodgkin lymphomas and related leukemias. Am. J. Path. 90:461-486, 1978.
2. Saltzstein, S.L.: Pulmonary malignant lymphomas and pseudo-lymphomas: Classification, therapy and prognosis. Cancer 16:928-955, 1963.

Malignant Lymphoma, Small Noncleaved Follicular Center Cell, Diffuse, Terminal Ileum

Clinical History

This 2½-year-old Mexican-American male was admitted on June 8, 1975, with a one-month history of colic epigastric pain, repeated emesis, mild anorexia and a 9 lb weight loss. During the day prior to admission, the epigastric pain became very severe, and he was unable to tolerate food. There was no previous gastrointestinal disorder. Physical examination indicated a scaphoid abdomen with a tender mobile and firm right upper quadrant mass, measuring 3 cm in diameter. The bowel sounds were normal and the rectal examination was normal except for a trace positive occult blood. No lymphadenopathy was detected. Laboratory data included a hematocrit of 28.2%, hemoglobin of 8.8 gm%, WBC of 13,000 cells/mm^3, platelets 550,000/mm^3 and an erythrocyte sedimentation rate of 30 mm/hr. A barium enema disclosed ileocolic intussusception with a probable lead point mass. On June 10, 1975, an exploratory laparotomy was performed, and a tumor was found in the terminal ileum, approximately 1.5 cm proximal to the ileocecal valve, which was the lead point mass, causing the ileocolic intussusception.

Gross Pathology

Thirteen centimeters of distal ileum and 6 cm of ascending colon with cecum and appendix were removed. The cut surface of the tumor was homogenous, yellow-tan tissue.

Microscopic Findings

In this specimen a primitive cellular proliferation extends from the mucosa beneath an ulcerated area through much of the intestinal wall. Despite multiple sections available for study, it is impossible to determine if the tumor extended entirely through the muscularis to the serosa. At the margin of the tumor with the intact mucosa, reactive follicles are present. Several ill-defined nodular areas, possibly lymphomatous follicles, are observed in the adjacent tissue. The process throughout the tumor otherwise is diffuse in character. Scattered irregularly throughout the tumor are numerous starry-sky phagocytes containing prominent nuclear debris. The primary tumor cell is intermediate in size with nuclear detail that is difficult to characterize due to poor fixation. Mitoses are numerous. Examination of this tumor demonstrates the problem of poor fixation and slow penetration of the formalin fixation in large masses. Multiple thin slices are required to achieve ideal fixation. The touch imprints of the specimen were obtained. They exhibit a moderate range in cell size and an intermixture of small lymphocytes. The tumor cells have finely dispersed acidophilic chromatin with striking nucleoli and prominent basophilic cytoplasm that contains a few small uniform-size vacuoles. The cytoplasm is strikingly pyroninophilic.

Special Studies

Cell suspensions were collected from the mass. Only 6% of the cells formed spontaneous E rosettes (T cells) while 100% of the cells marked with monospecific antiserum for IgM and none of the other heavy chains, and a similar proportion marked for lambda chain and none for kappa chains. The process is interpreted as a monoclonal IgM lambda type. The proportion of cells forming E rosettes does not indicate that some of the cells are double marking, but rather different aliquots of the specimen may contain a slight variation in the proportions of B and T cells.

	E	EAC	EA	PV	M	G	A	D	κ	λ
Bowel lesion	6	16	0	100	100	0	0	0	0	100
Bone marrow	49	1	0	23	21	0	0	0	22	23

Histologic Differential Diagnosis

The diagnoses to consider in this case are listed in Table 1.

Table 1. Differential Diagnosis

Ileocecal-Mesentery Mass

1. Small noncleaved FCC
   Burkitt's type
   Non-Burkitt's type
2. Granulocytic sarcoma
3. Immunoblastic reaction (pseudolymphoma)

The diagnosis and classification of lesions of the ileocecal valve region and mesentery usually are readily established as a small noncleaved FCC type. They are usually diffuse and only occasionally have some residual nodularity. The principal question is whether this lesion fulfills the criteria for a Burkitt lymphoma with nuclei of rather uniform size that are smaller than the histiocyte nucleus, or whether they are much more variable in size, have more prominent nucleoli and fall within the so-called non-Burkitt variant. In this case, the proliferation is smaller, more uniform and the nucleoli are not unduly prominent and closely approach a Burkitt lymphoma. In our experience, childhood lymphoma of the small noncleaved type present principally in the ileocecal valve region or mesentery and the remainder in the facial region either in the orbit, maxillary sinus or even nasopharynx and uncommonly in peripheral lymph nodes.

Also for consideration is a chloromatous mass which may present in the gastrointestinal tract and in the mesentery and a severe mesenteric lymphadenitis when it may be of striking severe immunoblastic type. Pseudolymphomas in general also deserve consideration, but these are principally lymphocytic and composed of small lymphocytes with a mixture of plasma cells and occasionally reactive follicles. In a child or young adult in the Mediterranean region, the diagnosis of alpha chain would deserve primary consideration [1]. Several of the cases reported by Ramot et al presented the morphologic features that resembled the Burkitt type [2]. This process, however, is associated with an intense plasma cell proliferation in the lamina propria that may extend throughout most of the small intestine.

Staging

This type of lymphoma involvement is difficult to evaluate meaningfully by current staging systems. This lymphoma was limited to the gastrointestinal tract and adjacent lymph nodes were negative. This is stage IIE by some criteria, but others recognize this staging sequence may not be adequate for abdominal extranodal lymphoma. A separate clinical staging system for Burkitt's lymphoma has been proposed [3].

Clinical Correlation and Follow-up

The patient is alive and well three years following resection. The small noncleaved FCC type in our experience predominantly has an abdominal presentation. In our series from the Childrens Hospital of Los Angeles (CHLA), 46 of 114 cases collected during a 25-year period (1950-1975) were of this type, and over 70% had an abdominal presentation [4]. The remainder were essentially from the facial region, either maxillary sinus or nasopharynx. In a separate study of lymphoma-leukemia in childhood during a two-year period, six examples of small noncleaved FCC lymphoma were noted in the series of 49 patients. The current case is Case 1 of Table 3 of the report [5]. Through the years we have observed many cases in children and young adults presenting with an ileocecal valve mass. This association of a B cell type with a mass infiltration in the lamina proprias strongly suggests that the lymphoma arises primarily in Peyer's patch type of lymphoid tissue and then spreads in a fashion parallel to a carcinoma. This consideration emphasizes the importance of clinical staging and also raises the potential of curability of processes that may be limited to the bowel wall. In his experience with a limited number of cases, Dr. Saul Rosenberg from Stanford University (personal communication) has indicated that children with lesions limited to the bowel wall without lymph node involvement have had disease-free survival and probable cures with only radiation therapy to the operative bed following resection. It seems likely that if these indeed are primary tumors that the prognosis relates to whether the lesion is limited to the bowel wall or involves mesenteric nodes. This consideration adds further evidence to the importance of careful staging at time of surgery. From our study of the series from the CHLA cases, it was apparent that over one third of the cases developed leukemic marrow involvement during the course of the disease and principally during relapse. Cytologically, the cells resemble those demonstrated in the imprints and may be included in acute lymphocytic leukemia, but will mark as the B cell type and have an entirely different prognosis from the so called null cell ALL.

In a review of 30 patients with Burkitt's lymphoma seen at the NCI, the abdomen was the most common site of involvement [6]. However, marrow involvement was noted in five cases.

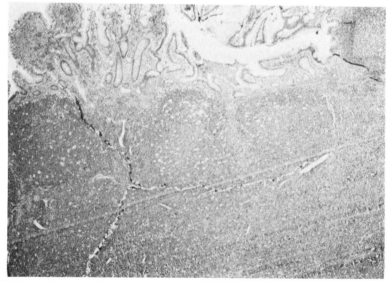

FIG. 1. Terminal ileum with diffuse proliferation of primitive cells with several areas suggestive of follicularity (nodularity) immediately beneath the epithelium (H & E 12.5×).

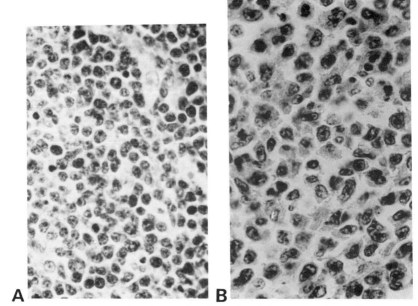

FIG. 2. Cellular proliferation varies throughout the tumor depending upon the penetration of the fixative (A). Centrally in the specimen, the cells appear loose, appear noncohesive, retracted cytoplasm (B) (H & E 125X). In the more superficial areas, the cells have more cytoplasm and are more cohesive. In both regions the cells vary somewhat in size and in configuration, often appearing slightly irregular as in B. Nuclear chromatin in both specimens is highly distributed but in this less than optimum fixation nucleoli are not well portrayed (H & E 500X).

References

1. Lewin, K.J., Kahn, L.B. and Novis, B.H.: Primary intestinal lymphoma of "Western" and "Mediterranean" type, alpha chain disease and massive plasma cell infiltration. A comparative study of 37 cases. Cancer 38:2511-2528, 1976.
2. Ramot, B. and Hulu, N.: Primary intestinal lymphoma and its relation to alpha heavy chain disease. Br. J. Cancer 31:343-349, 1975.
3. Ziegler, J.L.: Treatment. Results of 54 American patients with Burkitt's lymphoma are similar to the African experience. N. Engl. J. Med. 297:75-80, 1977.
4. Schneider, B.K., Higgens, G.R., Swanson, V. et al: Malignant lymphomas in childhood. Blood 46:1015, 1975.
5. Williams, A.H., Taylor, C.R., Higgins, G.R. et al: Childhood lymphoma-leukemia. I. Correlation of morphology and immunological studies. Cancer 42:171-181, 1978.
6. Arseneau, J.C., Canellos, G.P., Banks, P.M. et al: American Burkitt's lymphoma: A clinicopathologic study of 30 cases. I. Clinical factors relating to prolonged survival. Am. J. Med. 58:314-329, 1975.

Granulocytic Sarcoma, Orbital Mass

Clinical History

This 15-year-old male in Kenya had a mass in the peri-orbital region for an unknown length of time. Symptoms are not recorded and the laboratory findings indicated a hemo-globin of 12 gm and total white blood count of 8,000 cells/mm^3. The peripheral blood smear was not examined.

Gross Pathology

Not available.

Microscopic Findings

The specimen is a highly cellular infiltrative tumor without discernible architectural features or peripheral demarcations. The tumor cells extend into skeletal muscle and between the muscle fibers. In one section, there is a portion appearing to be eyelid with extension of tumor into the subepidermal loose connective tissue. The cellular infiltration is primitive in appearance and oriented to the connective tissue vascular structures. In the H & E stained sections there is no obvious cellular border or readily discernible cytoplasm. In most areas it is densely cellular without discernible "starry-sky" phago-cytes. On close inspection, the cells have generally round nuclei that are oval with a range in nuclear size. They have finely dispersed chromatin and usually a small centrally situ-ated nucleolus. Scattered throughout the cellular infiltrate are a few cells with definite eosinophilic granules. These eosino-philic cells are mononuclear and have nuclei of the same size range and configuration of those without eosinophil granules. These eosinophilic cells fulfill the criteria for eosinophilic myelocytes. Mitoses are readily identified, but they are not strikingly numerous. The tumor cells, while appearing primitive by their nuclear chromatin distribution, are relatively uniform in size and configuration and lack bizarreness of pleomorphic sarcoma. No multinucleated forms were noted.

Special Studies

The methyl green pyronine stain shows pyroninophilic cytoplasm. The eosinophilic component is dramatically obvious in Giemsa stained sections, and a number of the cells are strikingly positive in the immunoperoxidase stains for muramidase (lysozyme). A number of the cells are positive in the CAE (chloroacetate esterase stain) for granulocytes. It should be emphasized, however, that the original finding of eosinophilic myelocytes in the H & E stained section in my experience has proven a reliable indicator that the associated primitive cells are granulocytes, if the nuclear characteristics of the eosinophilic myelocyte and the tumor cells are similar.

Histologic Differential Diagnosis

The principal histologic differential diagnoses are (1) Burkitt lymphoma, (2) retinoblastoma, (3) rhabdomyosarcoma and (4) granulocytic sarcoma. In this case with an orbital presentation in a boy living in Kenya, the obvious clinical differential diagnosis is a Burkitt lymphoma and retinoblastoma. Incidentally, this specimen was submitted as an example of a Burkitt lymphoma diagnosed initially in Kenya. However, the pathologists were misled by the anatomic site combined with the frequency of an orbital or facial presentation of the Burkitt lymphoma. The cells of the Burkitt lymphoma, which we believe are of the small noncleaved follicular center cell (FCC) type, are also of intermediate size; they have nuclei smaller than the starry-sky histiocyte nucleus, finely dispersed chromatin and two or three small nucleoli frequently found distributed in an orderly, irregular fashion, often on the nuclear membrane. The cytoplasm is distinctly pyroninophilic and moderate in amount; in well-fixed specimens, the cytoplasmic borders are cohesive. Eosinophilic myelocytes are absent. A second possibility for orbital tumor in a child is embryonal rhabdomyosarcoma. This tumor is also primitive, but considerably more pleomorphic and has much more prominent mitotic activity. A third consideration is orbital retinoblastoma which accounted for 34.5% of 191 orbito-ocular tumors in Nigerians reported by Olurin and Williams [1]. The majority of these Nigerian tumors were poorly differentiated and only three cases showed rosettes. These three patients were older than usual (5, 7 and 8 years) and the older age of 15 years would be extremely unusual for retinoblastoma [1]. The MGP stain shows no cytoplasmic pyroninophilia although in Burkitt's lymphoma some positive cells should be seen. Another consideration is granulocytic sarcoma. For the general surgical pathologist who does not frequently examine the hematopoietic tissue in histologic sections commonly, the diagnosis of chloroma is difficult principally because it is a rare tumor and the possibility does not readily come to mind. Because of the primitive general features of chloroma, the process in general may resemble many poorly differentiated tumors, depending upon the anatomic site of involvement at presentation. From a cytologic standpoint, the features are distinctive and the associated eosinophilic myelocytes readily permit an accurate diagnosis. The tumor cells have round to oval nuclei that are considerably larger than the combined size of the normal two nuclei of a mature eosinophil. The CAE (chloroacetate esterase) cytochemical procedure provides a strong confirmation of the granulocyte nature of the proliferation.

Previous reports of orbital chloroma have been made, but in the large series of 191 orbital-ocular tumors in the Nigerian series, no diagnosis of chloroma was recorded. In the case of Gump et al, leukemia was present at the time of diagnosis of the orbital tumor [2]. A review of 166 leukemic children from Turkey revealed that 20 had orbital tumor [3]. All 20 children had acute myelomonocytic form and 17 had orbital onset before clinical recognition of leukemia. One patient was diagnosed eight months after eye involvement was noted.

Clinical Staging

Ordinarily in dealing with patients with granulocytic leukemia, the question of clinical staging does not arise, but in a patient with chloroma, clinical staging and restaging are of the utmost importance. It is essential to determine if the patient has marrow involvement in any approachable site. Usually when a chloroma is encountered, the marrow has already been involved and leukemic manifestations in the peripheral blood may already be evident. In a small proportion of the cases, a chloromatous mass is found and the marrow on examination is essentially normal and a lengthy interval may occur before leukemia develops. In this situation interval hematologic examinations and marrow examinations are required. Possibly chromosomal examinations of the marrows of these patients before leukemia development becomes apparent may serve as a useful guideline.

Clinical Correlation and Follow-up

Chloromas are composed essentially of myeloblasts and present in a wide variety of locations, but most commonly either as a destructive bone lesion or in association with bone. An orbital mass presentation, as in this case, possibly may have been an extension from an underlying bone lesion. In our personal experience, we have observed chloroma in the gastrointestinal tract, in the ovary, the breast and the thymus. Chloromas are usually found in patients with marrow evidence of granulocytic leukemia that is also of poorly differentiated or myeloblastic type, and the prognosis thus is of a poorly differentiated granulocytic leukemia. In a small proportion of the cases the chloroma precedes evidence of marrow involvement by a few months to two years [4]. Whether the chloromatous foci represent the initial focus of the leukemia or an exaggeration of the systemic process is unknown.

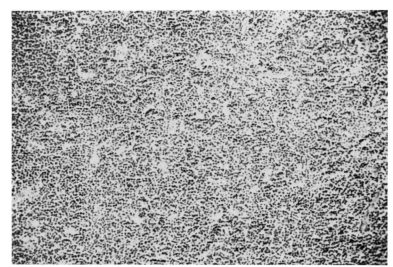

FIG. 1. Diffuse proliferation of primitive cells with scattered starry-sky phagocytes shown as lightly staining areas (H & E 50×).

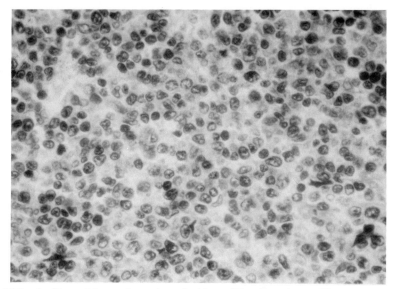

FIG. 2. Resemblance to a lymphoid proliferation is readily apparent. Though eosinophilic myelocytes were found in some areas, and the cloroacetate esterase stain revealed myelocytes and poorly differentiated granulocytes, they are impossible to portray properly in this black and white photomicrograph (H & E 500×).

References

1. Olurin. O. and Williams, A.O.: Orbito-occular tumors in Nigeria. Cancer 30.580-587, 1972.
2. Gump, M.E., Hester, E.G. and Lohr, O.W.: Monocytic chloroma (reticulocystoblastoma with monocytic leukemia). Arch. Ophthalmol. 16:931-949, 1936.
3. Cavdar, A., Arcasoy, A., Babacan, E. et al: Ocular granulocytic sarcoma (chloroma) with acute myelomonocytic leukemia in Turkish children. Cancer 41:1606-1609, 1978.
4. Mason, T.E., Demaree, R.S. Jr., and Margolis, C.I.: Granulocytic sarcoma (chloroma), two years preceding myelogenous leukemia. Cancer 31:423-432, 1973.

Malignant Lymphoma, Large Noncleaved Follicular Center Cell, Diffuse, Tonsil

Clinical History

This 75-year-old Mexican-American male was in good health until February 1974 when he noted difficulty in swallowing. He had lost approximately 25 lb in weight and coughed a small amount of bloody material. On physical examination, a fungating mass of the left hypopharynx was noted. Right submandibular nodes were nontender and slightly enlarged and on the left side of the neck there was a 3 X 4 cm nontender mass. A biopsy of February 7, 1974, revealed undifferentiated malignant tumor. Subsequently on March 11, 1974, the left tonsillar mass was excised.

Gross Pathology

The tumor measured 5.5 X 4 cm and was friable fishflesh tissue which had a mucosal lining on one surface. The cut surface shows focal necrosis and nodulation.

Microscopic Findings

This tonsillar specimen is partially covered by stratified squamous epithelium with areas of ulceration. The majority of the tonsil is replaced by amorphous proliferation of large cytoplasmic cells with an occasional peripheral reactive follicle. In one area, two follicles were found beneath the epithelium in which the follicular center cells were considered to be identical with the cells in the mass. These follicles are on a margin of the massive infiltration. The cytoplasmic tumor cells have large round to oval nuclei with finely dispersed chromatin with small nucleoli commonly situated on the nuclear membrane. The

49

cytoplasm is prominent, amphophilic and often the cellular borders are cohesive. In areas they occur in elongated clusters with fairly well-defined borders adjacent to small round lymphocytes. Mitoses are numerous. Examination of varying portions of the specimen at different depths reveals that there is a definite tendency for the cells to aggregate and these clusters are separated by lymphocytic infiltration.

The appearance of the nuclei varies considerably depending upon the quality of fixation. At times the nuclei are vesicular and devoid of nuclear chromatin because of delayed penetration of the specimen at this depth. The cytoplasm is intensively pyroninophilic in the most ideal fixed portions, and at times it is pale and less well defined in the deeper portions.

Special Studies

Cell suspensions were prepared on this case and immuno-logic surface marker studies performed. A monoclonal surface immunoglobulin of the IgM kappa type was demonstrated and presented further support for the interpretation of a malignant lymphoma in this case. This case demonstrates an additional value of the surface marker studies when there is a difficult differential diagnosis between carcinoma and malignant lymphoma.

Functional studies	E	EAC	EA	PV	M	G	A	D	κ	λ
	39	ND	ND	34	31	1	1	ND	16	0

Histologic Differential Diagnosis

The differential diagnosis of this lesion is (1) undif-ferentiated carcinoma and (2) malignant lymphoma of trans-formed lymphocytes, either a large noncleaved FCC or an immunoblastic sarcoma. The cohesive clusters of the tumor cells evident in many areas of the specimen cause considerable con-cern for the possibility of a carcinoma, but the resemblance of the cells to transformed lymphocytes provides strong support for the possibility of malignant lymphoma. The finding in one area of definite lymphomatous follicles finally provides conclu-sive evidence of the lymphomatous nature of this process.

Clinical Staging

The patient was subjected to the clinical staging with lymphangiography liver, spleen and bone marrow scans, gallium scans and examination of bone marrow in search of possible lymphomatous involvement. No evidence of disease was demonstrated and the patient was thus staged as clinical stage (CS) IIE_B.

Clinical Correlation and Follow-up

This case raises the question of the origin of malignant lymphoma in a tonsil, and the lack of evidence after thorough clinical staging procedures leaves little doubt that this is a primary lymphoma of the tonsil. The rapid widespread dissemination of the process fits well with the high turnover rate type of proliferation of the large noncleaved FCC type when it is not responsive to therapy. Lymphoma limited to the tonsil when it can be validated reasonably as a stage IE disease is of major prognostic significance with a high likelihood of curable disease. With extension of the disease to the adjacent lymph node as stage IIE the prognosis changes significantly, since it greatly heightens the possibility of disseminated disease at the time of initial diagnosis. In this case, the presence of a 25 lb weight loss as a prominent B symptom strongly indicated the likelihood that the disease had already disseminated, even though it was not detected by clinical staging procedures. Its rapid progression would seem to indicate a complete lack of responsiveness to chemotherapy.

Involvement of the tonsils in non-Hodgkin's lymphoma is relatively frequent and extremely rare in Hodgkin's disease (less than 1%) [1]. The incidence of tonsil involvement of non-Hodgkin's lymphoma may be common in some geographic areas as reported by Bonadonna et al from the National Cancer Institute in Milan, Italy, where 20% to 57% of adult patients presented with Waldeyer ring involvement. This observation suggests the possible geographic carcinogenic factor, but no studies thus far have been completed to elucidate this unusual finding. Interestingly, this patient had no gastrointestinal involvement recognized during relapse which is common with lymphoma arising in Waldeyer ring (20% within three years).

He received 2000 rads to the tonsillar beds in March 1974. Subsequently he was treated with combination chemotherapy COPP. He tolerated therapy poorly with a 20 lb weight loss. In August 1974, an abdominal nodule was noted and within several weeks multiple nodules were palpable. An abdominal nodule was biopsied and revealed lymphomatous infiltration that was identical with that described in tonsils. Cell suspensions were collected for immunologic surface marker studies and revealed a low level of cells with globulin (less than 40%), but there was monoclonal surface immunoglobulin of IgM kappa type. Inguinal lymph nodes were enlarged by September 1974 and additional chemotherapy was instituted. He received radiation therapy in December 1974 and developed diffuse pulmonary infiltrates detected by chest radiograph. He expired on May 3, 1975 (15 months after diagnosis) of intractable congestive heart failure secondary to widespread lymphoma.

An autopsy was performed two days after death and lymphoma was found in the subcutaneous tissue of the chest, as multiple small nodules (1 cm diameter) in the liver (1100 gm), within the spleen (110 gm), within multiple lymph nodes in the retroperitoneum, posterior mediastinum, and hilum of lung, and within the prostate. No lymphoma was detected within the anterior mediastinum, axillary lymph nodes or pulmonary parenchyma.

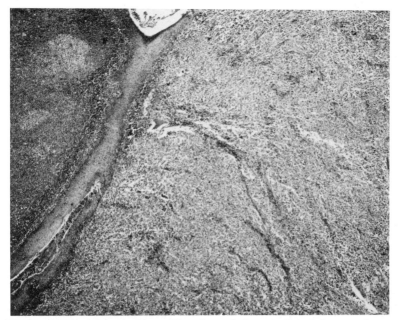

FIG. 1. Diffuse lymphoid proliferation of the tonsil is below an intact squamous epithelium (H & E 12.5×).

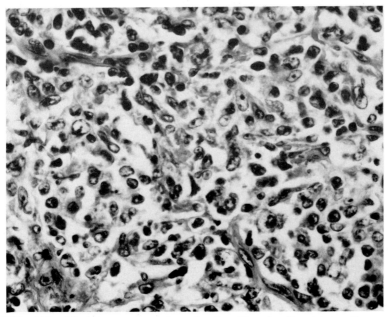

FIG. 2. Proliferation composed predominantly of cells with medium to large round oval nuclei with finely dispersed chromatin and one or two small nucleoli. There is a moderate amount of cytoplasm apparent in the noncohesive areas (H & E 500×).

Reference

1. Banti, A., Bonadonna, G., Carnevalli, G. et al: Lymphoreticular sarcomas with primary involvement of Waldeyer's ring. Cancer
   26:341-351, 1970.

Malignant Lymphoma, Large Noncleaved Follicular Center Cell, Minimally Follicular in Thyroid With Chronic Thyroiditis

Clinical History

This 44-year-old Caucasian female was admitted on December 7, 1975, for a rapidly enlarging right thyroid lump. She had a previous history of a small left thyroid nodule by palpation. The right lobe enlargement occurred over a 1½ week period and approximately 75% of the upper lobe was cold by thyroid scan. A right thyroid lobectomy and left lobe biopsy were performed.

Gross Pathology

The tissue weighed 26 gm and the gland was smooth, rubbery, homogenous tan with ill-defined yellowish foci. A calcified focus was present which measured 0.3 cm in greatest dimension.

Microscopic Findings

The specimen of the right lobe of the thyroid was exhaustively examined with the entire lobe blocked and sampled. There was wide variation in the appearance of the process. There are three appearances depending upon the portion of the specimen examined. In one portion the specimen is heavily infiltrated by small round lymphocytes that widely separate thyroid follicles, and in some areas there is also prominent sclerosis. In other areas, a pattern is a prominent lymphocytic follicular hyperplasia, which is reactive. Some follicles are large and ill-defined and in these regions there appears to be diffuse involvement of the gland by medium size lymphoid elements with the features of transformed lymphocytes. These lympho-

55

cytes present the features of noncleaved FCC. Even within these areas there is considerable variation in the cellular proliferation. A third pattern is the change in the thyroid epithelium of the thyroid follicles scattered throughout the gland. There is prominent epithelial proliferation with dysplasia which appears squamous. In one section a small papillary adenocarcinoma of thyroid is noted.

Special Studies

Functional studies were not obtained. Immunoperoxidase studies indicated polyclonal staining in plasma cells and some cells were positive for muramidase.

Histologic Differential Diagnosis

The principal diagnostic problem is whether the abnormal lymphoid proliferation encountered is simply an expression of the extreme reaction that may be found in chronic thyroiditis or if lymphoma is present. Once again, this distinction depends critically upon ideal fixation in order to evaluate the cytologic details of lymphocytes. Follicular hyperplasia of lymphocytes may be prominent and even severe in thyroiditis and the lymphocytic follicles may be extremely large and irregular. The diagnosis of malignant lymphoma depends upon finding a predominance of cleaved FCC (either small or large) or noncleaved FCC. This is an example of noncleaved FCC-type malignant lymphoma. If the noncleaved FCC (the dividing cells) of the follicular center are predominant, usually the margins of the follicles are not discernible and the process extends throughout the gland. This feature of the process appears to be the result of a rapidly proliferating cell, such as the noncleaved FCC cell, and it rapidly extends throughout the gland. Thus, the process changes from follicular to diffuse.

Clinical Staging

This patient was evaluated in great detail with noninvasive procedures, but no evidence of disease was found.

As part of the therapeutic approach, a decision was made to remove the remaining left lobe of the thyroid and search for lymph nodes on both sides of the neck. The remaining left lobe of thyroid was heavily infiltrated by lymphocytes and numerous reactive plasma cells without any evidence of follicular hyperplasia or malignant lymphoma. The total specimen was blocked and examined. No enlarged lymph nodes were found and the several nodes sampled did not reveal any evidence of metastatic carcinoma or malignant lymphoma. After this exhaustive evaluation the patient was considered to have pathological stage I disease.

Clinical Correlation and Follow-up

The patient was not radiated and was doing well as of November 1978 (approximately three years after diagnosis. Serum immunoelectrophoresis, and bone marrow biopsy and aspiration were normal. The development of malignant lymphoma in the thyroid is uncommon and from our experience essentially occurs in long standing thyroiditis of various types. The development of lymphoma in this situation is parallel to the occurrence of lymphomas in a variety of abnormal immune processes described elsewhere in which immunoblastic sarcoma may develop from an abnormal immune reaction. The majority of cases we have encountered have been of immunoblastic sarcoma type, though it is understandable that a large non-cleaved FCC type noted in this case may occur when the immune reaction has a chronic follicular component. In the recent report of Burke, Butler and Fuller all but one of the 35 cases presented features of lymphomas of transformed lymphocytes [1]. In their study, it is interesting that in all 27 cases with residual thyroid tissue, lymphocytic thyroiditis was present and provided further evidence of the development of the lymphomas in abnormal immune proliferations. The prognosis in patients with thyroid involvement of malignant lymphoma depends upon whether the lymphoma is primary in the thyroid and if it is limited to the thyroid. This is an important consideration, since the thyroid may be involved secondarily from adjacent lymph nodes by direct extension in which case the thyroid is usually otherwise normal and lacks evidence of lymphocytic thyroiditis. Of considerable importance in this case is whether there is undetected microscopic spread beyond the region of the thyroid that may be the source of clinical recurrence and thus produce progressive disease. The importance of spread beyond the thyroid is dramatically demonstrated also in the report by Burke, Butler and Fuller in which 25% of their cases with disease that seemed to be confined to the thyroid actually progressed and the patients failed to survive beyond two years. However, the remaining patients continued to survive beyond ten years.

Reference

1. Burke, J.S., Butler, J.J. and Fuller, L.M.: Malignant lymphomas of the thyroid. A clinical pathologic study of 35 patients including ultra-structural observations. Cancer 39:1578-1602, 1977.

II
Immunoblastic Sarcoma

Introduction

A malignant lymphoma termed immunoblastic sarcoma (IBS) was described in the classification system of Lukes and Collins [1,2]. This lymphoma consists of a monomorphous proliferation of transformed lymphocytes. The clinical description of a large patient group had previously not been recorded until the recent series by Lichtenstein, Levine, Lukes et al [3]. The following is a short summary of that paper which includes more specific clinical information on each patient in the series of 33. Thirty percent of the 33 patients had a history of prior immune deficiency disease or malignant lymphoproliferative disease. Diffuse hypergammaglobulinemia was recorded in 44% of the patients tested. The clinical stage at the time of diagnosis resulted in stage I or II in 30%, whereas stages III and IV were recorded for 70%. Nearly one half of the patients had systemic symptoms at presentation and the median survival was 14 months. More rapid progression of disease and death was noted in patients with advance stage of disease, lymphopenia, and systemic symptoms.

The patient records were collected through review of the consultative service of Robert J. Lukes, M.D. Although 47 patients were subjected to review, 14 were reclassified as lymphocyte depletion Hodgkin's disease — 2 cases; Ewing's sarcoma — 1 case; and follicular center cell lymphoma — 11 cases. The criteria for inclusion in the study were based on histologic finding alone. These histologic criteria of IBS are the observation of a monomorphous proliferation of large cells having nuclei equal in size or greater than the nucleus of a reactive histiocyte. The nuclear membrane is regular and the chromatin finely distributed and pale staining. Often, two or three nuclei are prominent. In the B cell derived IBS, the cytoplasm is amphophilic on hematoxylin and eosin staining and strongly pyroninophilic when stained with methyl green pyronine. The T cell derived immunoblastic sarcoma has pale staining cytoplasm that is lightly pyroninophilic. The B cell IBS often demonstrates plasmacytoid features of the cytoplasm.

In Table 1 the sex and age breakdown is recorded.

Table 1. Patient Description

Sex	Age (Years)	Range (Years)
19 males	48.7	21-69
14 females	65	17-85

The females tended to be older than the males with IBS. The overall age range was 55.6 years. The location of the diagnostic area of these 33 patients is noted in Table 2.

Table 2. Location of IBS

Nodal:		
Generalized		11
Mediastinal and local		5
Local		7
	Total	23
Extranodal:		
Lung		4
GI		3
Testis		1
Skin		1
Marrow		1
	Total	10

Ten patients demonstrated extranodal disease with the lung being the most common site. Eleven of the 33 patients (48%) had generalized lymphadenopathy. Mediastinal involvement was noted in five patients who also had palpable axillary or cervical adenopathy. Seven other patients had localized lymphadenopathy in the neck or groin. The initial histologic interpretation of the tissues removed in these 33 patients was widely variable as indicated in Table 3.

More than half of the patients carried a diagnosis other than IBS. Histiocytic lymphoma was the most common classification as IBS is one of five lymphoma types recognized

Table 3. Referral Diagnosis: IBS

Immunoblastic sarcoma	14
Histiocytic lymphoma	11
Mixed lymphoma	1
Hodgkin's disease	4
Anaplastic carcinoma	1
Eosinophilic granuloma	1
Lymphoproliferative disorder	1

by the Lukes' and Collins' classification that fit into the histiocytic category of Rappaport.

The previous history of the patients indicated a previous immunologic anomaly in ten (30%) of the patients. Several patients developed IBS in association with other malignant lymphoproliferative disorders. IBS was recognized 24 months to 14 years following the diagnosis of these various malignancies. On the other hand, a benign lymphoproliferative anomaly was also associated with the development of IBS (Table 4).

The clinical stage of these patients was not systemically evaluated, but the records available indicate that 49% of the patients had systemic symptoms including fever, night sweats, weight loss and, in one instance, phlebitis. The clinical stage of the patients is recorded in Table 5.

Note that 70% of the patients were stage III or IV. Staging laparotomy in three patients led to reclassification of one

Table 4. Lymphoproliferative Disorders
Associated with IBS

Malignant:	
Lymphoma	1
Hodgkin's disease	1
Macroglobulinemia	1
CLL	1
Benign:	
Chronic	2
Celiac disease	1
Asthma	1
Rheumatoid arthritis	
with Sjogren's syndrome	1
Immunoblastic	
lymphadenopathy	1

Table 5. Initial Stage: IBS

Stage I	7
Stage II	3
Stage III	9
Stage IV	14

patient from stage II to stage III-S. Laboratory data indicated anemia present in 73% at the time of diagnosis. Thrombocytopenia was unusual as was granulocytopenia. However, 15 patients demonstrated peripheral lymphocyte counts less than $1000/mm^3$. Serum immunoglobulin levels were measured in 25 patients and monoclonal serum protein demonstrated in two. Eleven of 25 patients demonstrated polyclonal hypergammaglobulinemia. Quantitative immunglobulin levels indicated IgA elevation in six.

Therapy of this disease was difficult to evaluate in the 33 patients since the treatment varied widely. Twenty-seven patients received chemotherapy and 15 were given aggressive combination chemotherapy consisting of cyclophosphamide, vincristine, prednisone and procarbazine (COPP), or a modification of bleomycin, adriamycin, cyclophosphamide, vincristine and prednisone (BACOP). Less aggressive chemotherapy was given to eight patients. No uniform response was reported in either the group treated with aggressive chemotherapy or those given less aggressive chemotherapy. Radiation therapy was given to four patients with stage I disease. The variation in response of these several groups of patients varied from no response and death within months to partial remission or to no evidence of disease 24 months later. The median survival was 14 months. The extent of disease influenced survival as patients with localized disease did better than the 23 patients with disseminated disease who had a median survival of 5 months. Furthermore, systemic symptoms and lymphopenia at the time of diagnosis also correlated with poor survival. The classification of IBS into B or T lymphocyte cell origin also correlated with survival. Of the 20 patients with IBS of B cell origin, a shorter survival was noted than in 13 patients with T cell derived immunoblastic sarcoma.

The literature contains brief descriptions of IBS although frequently under an alternative term. A review of the litera-

Table 6. IBS Associated Diseases Previously Reported

Renal transplantation
Immunoblastic lymphadenopathy
Chronic thyroiditis
Sjogren's syndrome
Celiac disease
Alpha chain disease
Hashimoto's thyroiditis
Chronic lymphocytic leukemia

ture for the occurrence of malignant lymphoma in association with a variety of other diseases indicates that most of these associations may be IBS with a disease of prolonged immunologic abnormality. These diseases are tabulated in Table 6 and referenced in the article by Lichtenstein.

References

1. Lukes, R.J. and Collins, R.D.: Immunologic characterization of human malignant lymphomas. Cancer 34:1488-1503, 1974.
2. Lukes, R.J. and Collins, R.D.: New approaches to the classification of the lymphomata. Br. J. Cancer 31 (Suppl. 2):1-28, 1975.
3. Lichtenstein, A., Levine, A.M., Lukes, R.J. et al: Immunoblastic sarcoma. Cancer 43:343-352, 1979.

Malignant Lymphoma, Immunoblastic Sarcoma, B Cell, Spleen

Clinical History

This 38-year-old Mexican-American male was transferred from another hospital on March 3, 1976, for chemotherapy of "metastatic adenocarcinoma" of the lung. The patient noted gradual onset of malaise, anorexia, 15 lb weight loss and nonproductive cough. He experienced occasional night sweats with chills and fever. He had been a drug user for 20 years. While in custody at a rehabilitation center, a routine chest x-ray revealed a noncalcified irregular mass in the left upper lobe of the lung. A thoracotomy and left upper lobectomy on January 3, 1976, indicated an "undifferentiated carcinoma." He received Cobalt 60 radiation. Following transfer for further therapy, a liver spleen scan indicated multiple defects in the spleen. A bipedal lymphangiogram showed positive periaortic lymph nodes. In 1961 he had a positive VDRL and a positive FTA for which penicillin therapy was administered.

Laboratory data included a hemoglobin of 12.9 gm% and a WBC of 7900. Bone marrow aspiration showed no evidence of tumor and serum immunoglobulin indicated the IgG was 1450 ml (600-2000 mg%). IgA was 195 ml% (50-400 mg%) and IgM 390 ml (40-250 mg).

On April 8, 1976, a staging laparotomy with splenectomy, liver biopsy, bone biopsy and periaortic lymph node biopsy was performed. There was tumor involvement of the spleen, pancreas, stomach and retroperitoneum.

Gross Pathology

The spleen weight was enlarged but not weighed and measured 5.0 × 4.5 × 4.0 cm. The cut surface showed two bulging lobules with an intervening normal splenic parenchyma. The largest of the nodules was 4.2 × 3.4 cm.

Microscopic Findings

The tumors in the spleen and retroperitoneal nodes appeared similar. There was massive replacement of splenic and lymph node architecture without any residual discernible normal features. The tumor was sharply delimited from the residual splenic parenchyma. Large ill-defined areas of necrosis within both tissues (spleen and retroperitoneum) and numerous necrobiotic cells were scattered throughout all areas of the tumor. In the spleen, thin-walled dilated vascular channels within the necrotic areas were surrounded by zones of variable tumor cells. On higher magnification the cellular proliferation was recognized as medium-sized primitive appearing cells of irregular configuration with abundant cytoplasm and numerous mitotic figures. The nuclei had finely dispersed chromatin and nucleoli are small or inconspicuous. An occasional cell had a large nucleolus. Small nucleoli were observed on the nuclear membranes. The cytoplasm was confluent without well-defined cellular borders. Shrunken nuclei of necrotic cells were common. Frequently, nuclei were irregular because of deep indentations or nuclear cleaves and a few of the cells fulfill the criteria for large cleaved follicular center cells. Some areas of deeply staining cytoplasm suggest plasmacytoid features. Review of the lung lesion revealed the same tumor.

Special Studies

Immunoperoxidase studies for cytoplasmic immunoglobulin revealed a monoclonal type of immunoglobulin staining only for IgM heavy chain and kappa light chain. There was no evidence of the other heavy or light chains. Approximately 35% of the cells stained with this procedure. Many cells are lightly stained and a significant portion of the population did not appear to contain immunoglobulin.

A similar procedure for muramidase (lysozyme) failed to reveal any evidence of this histiocyte-monocyte enzyme. The ultrastructural studies of the specimens revealed that many cells were degenerating, but the discernible features in the intact cells were those of transformed lymphocytes without any evidence to suggest histiocytes or carcinoma. Numerous polyribosomes were seen without a significant amount of rough endoplasmic reticulum.

Immunologic surface marker studies were performed on cell suspensions prepared from both the tumor within the spleen and the retroperitoneal region. The findings in both specimens were identical with monoclonal marking of IgM kappa indicating B lymphocyte origin. In both specimens, over 80% of the cells have a single type of immunoglobulin which is the heavy chain IgM and the light chain kappa. The presence of a single type of immunoglobulin on the surface that is a monoclonal type is considered conclusive evidence of monoclonal origin from the B lymphocyte.

	E	EAC	EA	PV	M	G	A	D	κ	λ
Lymph node	4	0	0	91	82	0	0	0	90	0
Spleen	5	1	1	86	80	3	0	0	84	0

Histologic Differential Diagnosis

For decades cases of this histologic type have presented pathologists with great difficulty in precise diagnosis. Pathologists have resolved the diagnostic dilemma using the term reticulum cell sarcoma. This term has been shown to be of limited meaning and more recently associated with the histiocytic type of Rappaport. Our special studies clearly demonstrate that carcinoma can be excluded, although without the advantage of these procedures in other cases, this differentiation may be difficult unless optimum histologic material is available. It is now apparent from our multiparameter studies and those of others that most lymphomas of large cell type previously included as Rappaport's histiocytic type are not truly derived from histiocytes, but are transformed lymphocytes of either T or B type. The cytologic features provide clear evidence of a high turnover rate type of proliferation with numerous mitoses and cells that resemble transformed lymphocytes. The surface marker studies exclude histiocytic lymphoma because of the lack in the nonspecific esterase (a phagocytic enzyme) and muramidase (histiocyte-monocyte enzyme). The cells have the monoclonal surface immunoglobulin of the B cell; thus, final diagnosis with the help of these techniques rests between a large cleaved FCC lymphoma, a large noncleaved lymphoma and an immunoblastic sarcoma of B cells. In this case, the large cleaved FCC type can be excluded because the process principally is of a transformed lymphocytic type (without cleaved nuclei) even though a small number of the nuclei have deep cleavage planes. In our original evaluation of this case, it was our impression that some of the cells, especially in the spleen, exhibited plasma-cytoid features. For these reasons, it was classified as an im-munoblastic sarcoma of B cell type. At the time of conference presentation, and after preparation of sections from many blocks, we realized that "plasmacytoid component" was very limited, and the proliferation appears to fit better with the large noncleaved FCC type. This case clearly demonstrates the prob-lem in differential diagnosis between this cell type and the immunoblastic sarcoma. This distinction may be of therapeutic and prognostic significance. The cells of immunoblastic sarcoma have thicker nuclear membranes, more prominent nucleoli, denser and more amphophilic cytoplasm and appear to be a much more abnormal type of proliferation. From our pre-liminary kinetic studies of IBS it appears that the DNA content is extremely variable and even rather bizarre, and this may account for its general rapid progression and less favorable response to therapy. The large noncleaved cell type has some degree of follicle formation (approximately 10%) and at times retains some of the nuclear cleavage, even in the larger cells or may have a residual small cleaved cell component in which the nuclear membranes are thin, the chromatin more finely dispersed and the nucleoli small.

Clinical Staging

The clinical and laparotomy findings indicate pathologic stage IVB.

Clinical Correlation and Follow-up

Immunoblastic sarcoma and large NC FCC lymphoma may present as extranodal masses in unusual locations and resemble a carcinoma at times. These disorders may present in an abnormal immune state commonly and in this patient, a known drug addict of long duration, may have been exposed to chronic antigenic stimulation. At the present time (1979), it is undetermined whether drug addiction is associated with an increased incidence of lymphomas.

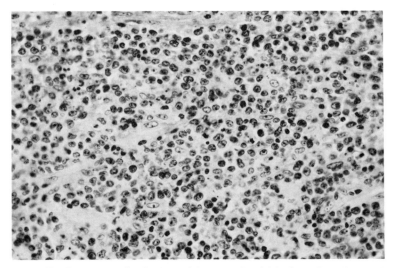

FIG. 1. Replacement of splenic architecture by fairly large lymphocytoid cells (H & E 125X).

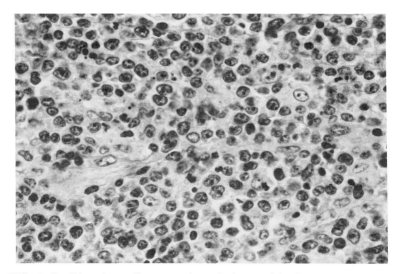

FIG. 2. Proliferating cells are moderately large with abundant cytoplasm and a nuclei showing dispersed chromatin with occasional prominent nucleoli (H & E 500×).

Malignant Lymphoma, Immunoblastic Sarcoma, Probably B Cell, Axillary Lymph Node

Clinical History

This 61-year-old nurse was seen at Mount Sinai Hospital in New York in 1951 for Sjogren's disease of the right parotid gland. Subsequently, a parotid biopsy was interpreted as Warthin's tumor and radiation therpy was administered. At the same time, a diagnosis of systemic lupus erythematosus was made and steroids were administered. In the family history, it was noted that the mother died of breast carcinoma and four brothers had hemophilia. The patient had a breast lump noted in May 1976 and a biopsy revealed in situ duct adenocarcinoma. On May 3, 1976, a simple mastectomy with axillary dissection of enlarged lymph nodes was performed.

Gross Pathology

Multiple soft pink-tan lymph nodes from the axilla measured 6 × 4 cm in diameter.

Microscopic Findings

The lymph node architecture was markedly altered by a proliferation of large cytoplasmic cells that extended throughout the node isolating small areas composed of lymphocytes leaving only an occasional subcapsular or medullary area in which the sinusoids were discernible. In the small portion of capsule available for review, penetration by these large cells was noted. The cytoplasmic cells varied moderately in size and had cohesive interlocking often well-demarcated borders. There was a range of nuclear size with the component of larger cells having nuclear features closely resembling those of transformed lymphocytes with round to oval configuration,

two to three prominent nucleoli and finely dispersed chromatin. The cytoplasm was usually pale staining. A small component of larger cytoplasmic cells had dense amphophilic
cytoplasm that suggested plasmacytoid origin. Mitoses were
numerous. With the methyl green pyronine stain, the cytoplasm of the pale cells was slightly positive, while those cells
with the amphophilic cytoplasm had intensely pyroninophilic
staining. The residual lymphocytes were small, irregular and
had scanty cytoplasm.

The distribution of the process in lymph node super-
ficially suggested a sinusoidal pattern, but on closer inspection, it was a confluent multifocal involvement leaving small
foci of lymphoid tissue. The residual sinusoids contained small
numbers of these cells.

Special Studies

The immunoperoxidase studies for cytoplasmic immunoglobulin and muramidase were extremely helpful. The cells
that appeared to have amphophilic cytoplasm stained in a
monoclonal fashion for kappa light chains and the heavy
chain IgA with only a small amount of staining with IgG. This
finding of the monoclonal cytoplasmic immunoglobulin provides support of the B cell nature of these cells. These cells
are plasmacytoid and this is similar to the plasmacytoid
features of some immunoblasts. The immunoperoxidase stain
for muramidase stained scattered cells other than the large
cytoplasmic cells which resembled immunoblasts. The special
studies thus provide support for the interpretation of the cells
as immunoblasts of B cell type.

Histologic Differential Diagnosis

This lymph node lesion presents an extraordinary appearance and presents considerable difficulty in diagnosis and,
therefore, a long differential diagnostic list (Table 1).

The multifocal involvement appearing to be a sinusoidal
pattern definitely raises the question of a metastatic process,
as does the prominent cytoplasmic feature of the large cell.
The occurrence of the patient with a carcinoma of the breast
and associated axillary lymph nodes must have caused con-

Table 1. Differential Diagnosis

1. Metastatic carcinoma
Breast (medullary?)
2. Metastatic melanoma
3. Malignant lymphoma
Histiocytic?

siderable problems for the original pathologist, had he not been such an astute observer. Fortunately, the original pathologist carefully collected and fixed the specimen ideally and it was possible to study the cytologic details in an excellently prepared specimen. It is easy to appreciate how impossible the correct diagnosis might have been on poorly collected material. The cohesive cytoplasmic character of these large cells brings to mind metastatic medullary carcinoma from the breast and metastatic amelanotic melanoma. The differentiation depends upon the identification of specific cytologic types. Specific techniques also permit precise cytologic characterization. In this case, the lack of muramidase staining makes the possibility of a histiocytic lymphoma unlikely and the presence of monoclonal cytoplasmic immunoglobulin conclusively establishing the B lymphocytic origin.

The differential diagnosis of the lymphoid lesions is not entirely simple. In the large cell group there appears to be five types previously included in the histiocytic lymphoma of Rappaport (Table 2).

The large cleaved cell can readily be excluded on the basis of its marked irregularity in nuclear configuration, the limited amount of cytoplasm and the frequent association with sclerosis. Often it exhibits marked polypoid cellular features. The true histiocytic in the limited number of cases studied thus far appears to have a range of expressions from monocyte to a plump cytoplasmic histiocyte and even an association with

Table 2. Histiocytic Lymphoma (Rappaport)

1. IBS − T cell
2. IBS − B cell
3. Large noncleaved FCC
4. Large cleaved FCC
5. True histiocytic

elongated spindle or fibroblastic component. Precise diagnosis at the present time requires specific cytochemical and anti-muramidase procedures. The remaining three categories of transformed lymphocytes derived lymphoma require considerable experience and excellent tissue preparation for distinction as proven in Case 21. The large noncleaved has a limited amount of pale staining cytoplasm that is prominent pyroninophilic and nuclei that have finely dispersed chromatin with several small nucleoli on the nuclear membrane.

The IBS B cell type has abundant cytoplasm that is usually intensely pyroninophilic and often is plasmacytoid to some degree. The IBS of T cell type has prominent abundant pale staining cytoplasm often appearing water-clear, well-demarcated cellular borders often arranged in interlocking fashion and usually a range of nuclear size. The nuclear features of individual cells in the T and B cell type at the present time appear similar. The immunoperoxidase studies for cytoplasmic immunoglobulin and the surface immunologic markers are needed at present to make the distinction, but in the future it may be possible to distinguish the T or B origin on morphologic grounds together with the immunoperoxidase studies for cytoplasmic immunoglobulin. Therefore, paraffin embedded tissue rather than functional studies on fresh tissue may be utilized for classification.

Clinical Correlation and Follow-up

This patient died with disseminated disease in lymph nodes approximately 16 months after diagnosis. The association of Sjogren's disease with the development of malignant lymphomas has been known since the report to Talal et al [1-3]. Furthermore, recently it has been demonstrated that Sjogren's disease has a genetic association with an HLA type (B8-Dw3) [4]. A large number of autoimmune disorders have been associated with HLA-B8 and this is further support for the concept of an abnormal immune response leading to malignant disorder of transformed lymphocytes. This case illustrates the development of immunoblastic sarcoma in an abnormal immune disorder. According to our concept, a switch-on of the lymphocyte transformation mechanism in a defective immune system may produce malignant lymphoma. In our experience, the immunoblastic sarcomas of this type are always of B cell type. The basic question in this situation relates to the reason for the loss of the control mechanism of lymphocyte transformation and the reason for occurrence in the seventh decade. A second question is, did the alteration in the T cell control mechanism of B cell transformation relate to the development of the breast carcinoma in this patient? The development of lymphoma in a patient with Sjogren's disease may occur in the salivary gland area or in any lymphoid tissue region because the patient has a fundamentally abnormal immune system. We have few examples of carcinoma development in lymphoma patients, but further critical review of this association is needed.

The association of Sjogren's syndrome and SLE has also been recognized [5]. Steinberg and Talal presented eight patients with this combination and hypergammaglobulinemia was common. The SLE abnormal immune function may be present as indicated by the various antibodies formed, but malignant lymphoma has not been a recognized sequelae in very many patients.

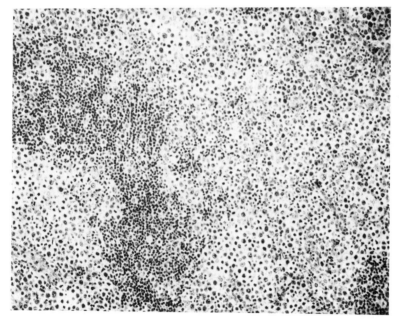

FIG. 1. Lymph node architecture is distorted by large cells with no residual follicles noted (H & E 125×).

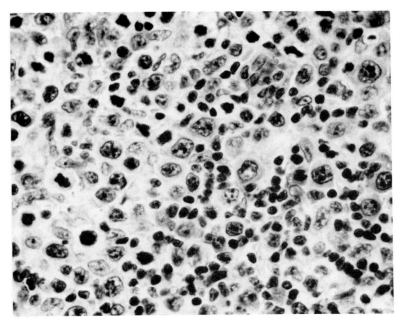

FIG. 2. Large cells have round to oval nuclei, several prominent nucleoli and finely dispersed chromatin. The cytoplasm is pale and there is a small number of residual lymphocytes scattered (H & E 500×).

References

1. Talal, N. and Bunim, J.J.: The development of malignant lymphoma in the course of Sjogren's syndrome. Am. J. Med. 36:529-540, 1964.
2. Talal, N., Sokoloff, L. and Barth, W.F.: Extrasalivary lymphoid abnormalities in Sjogren's syndrome (reticulum cell sarcoma, "pseudolymphoma," macroglobinemia). Am. J. Med. 43:50-65, 1967.
3. Zulman, J., Jaffe, R. and Talal, N.: Evidence that the malignant lymphoma of Sjogren's syndrome is a monoclonal B-cell neoplasm. N. Engl. J. Med. 299:1215-1220, 1978.
4. Chused, T.M., Kassan, S.S., Opelz, G. et al: Sjogren's syndrome associated with HLA Dw3. N. Engl. J. Med. 296:895-897, 1977.
5. Steinberg, A.D. and Talal, N.: The coexistence of Sjogren's syndrome and systemic lupus erythematosus. Ann. Intern. Med. 74:55-61, 1971.

Malignant Lymphoma, Immunoblastic Sarcoma, Plasmacytoid, B Cell Type, Mass Right Posterior Thorax

Clinical History

This 52-year-old Caucasian male noted intrascapular pain during a routine physical examination. The pain increased but remained localized without radiation to other areas. There were no systemic symptoms. A chest radiograph showed a right posterior mediastinal mass measuring 6.5 × 4.0 cm lying in the paravertebral gutter and no bone alterations were noted. An excision of the thoracic mass was completed on March 17, 1976.

Gross Pathology

The numerous tissue fragments measured up to 6.5 cm and weighed a total of 37 gm. Some fragments were friable and slightly pink whereas other areas showed hemorrhage and a shaggy membrane. The cut surface revealed bulging uniformly pink-orange tissue with some suggestion of fibrous septae.

Microscopic Findings

The specimen was soft tissue infiltrated by plasmacytoid cells of varying size and appearance. The infiltration extended around the vessels but not into them. No discernible evidence of lymph node architecture was noted. The tumor cells varied considerably in size with the nuclei ranging from a small lymphocyte size to that of a fully transformed lymphocyte. The larger cells had features of transformed lymphocytes or immunoblasts with finely dispersed chromatin and two to

79

three nucleoli of uniform size often distributed in a uniform fashion. The cytoplasm was strikingly amphophilic and commonly appeared plasmacytoid and a number of the cells had a distinctive "hof." The amount of cytoplasm also varied widely and was prominent in those cells that stained intensively amphophilic and possessed the "hof." A large proportion of the population had a limited amount of cytoplasm with a central nucleus rather than eccentric as in plasmacytoid cells. Many of the cells had the appearance of medium-sized transformed lymphocytes with round nuclei and finely dispersed chromatin and often a single central nucleolus. The cells were arranged in closely packed frequently cohesive masses. In the methyl green pyronine stain, the degree of pyroninophilia varied considerably apparently as a result of differences in fixation; cells presenting a cytoplasmic hof were most apparent in this stain and were numerous. Distributed throughout the specimen were variable numbers of large cells with pleomorphic features and nuclei that were extremely large or even binucleated. These cells appeared to be extremely atypical immunoblasts. Mitoses were common and thus the tumor cells were variable in morphology with many variations of cytoplasmic and nuclear features of transformed lymphocytes.

Special Studies

The immunoperoxidase studies for cytoplasmic immunoglobulin and muramidase were extremely revealing. In the majority of cells the cytoplasm contains striking amounts of monoclonal IgA kappa chain and a small proportion of the cells are negative. Scattered cells of monocytoid or histiocyte character were positive for muramidase and widely scattered throughout the process.

Histologic Differential Diagnosis

The prominent plasmacytoid features of this process raise the question of three possibilities: (1) a plasmacytoma, (2) an extramedullary myeloma and (3) an immunoblastic sarcoma B cell type with plasmacytoid features. The term plasmacytoma has been applied in a variable fashion depending upon the anatomic region. Often it has been used by a pathologist uncertain about the prognosis of an abnormal plasma cell proliferation, particularly for tumors in the nose and nasopharynx where extensive plasma cell proliferations may be prominent. From our experience, these proliferations exhibit features of reactive plasma cells which are excessive in number. Such proliferations contain benign appearing plasma cells of varying size without their precursor cells which are the immunoblasts. The second possibility, extramedullary myeloma, in our view can be readily discounted on both morphologic and clinical grounds. Myeloma is a uniform proliferation of abnormal plasma cells. The myeloma cell has distinctive abnormal plasma cell features with the entire population exhibiting the same level of nuclear maturation, though the nuclei may vary somewhat in size. The cytoplasm varies in amount, but is consistently plasmacytoid in all cells. Occasionally in myeloma the process may change to a proliferation of its precursors the immunoblasts, but a separate population of these cells develops as a distinctive component rather than intermingled as individual cells. When the latter situation develops, it has been designated multiple myeloma with reticulum cell sarcoma. In reality, we believe the situation represents a change in myeloma to immunoblastic sarcoma, as a result of the switch on the lymphocyte transformation mechanism. In this case the monoclonal cytoplasmic immunoglobulin of IgA type demonstrates the neoplastic and monoclonal character of the cellular proliferation. IgA is found at types in myeloma, but infrequently (5% to 10%). Clinically, myeloma seems unlikely in a patient without detectable bone lesions, significant monoclonal serum immunoglobulin abnormality, or easily recognized plasma cells. This process in our case represents a malignant lymphoma called immunoblastic sarcoma and has features of relatively mature functioning plasma cells. It is considered to be a lymphoma since the significant component of the process appears to be medium- to large-sized transformed lymphocytes with minor degrees of plasmacytoid features. The process is also infiltrative and aggressive, can be readily distinguished from a benign accumulation of reactive plasma cells. The monoclonicity of the cytoplasmic immunoglobulin provides essentially conclusive evidence of their neoplastic nature. If malignant lymphoma is considered and the Rappaport classification is utilized, there is no ideal category unless the term histiocytic lymphoma with plasmacytoid feature is used. This is analogous to a term that has been used in the literature: plasmacytoid reticulum cell sarcoma.

Clinical Staging

A bone survey was normal and bone marrow showed 7% plasma cells. Therefore, this is pathologic stage I.

Clinical Correlation and Follow-up

This is considered an example of mediastinal IBS and these patients usually have palpable (localized) lymphadenopathy. The posterior location suggests this is arising in lymph node. Serum immunoglobulin levels were frequently altered as reported in our series of 33 patients with IBS. In this patient, the IgA was slightly increased and there was a slight decrease in IgG and IgM. He received six weeks of radiation therapy. Nineteen months later he died with diffuse metastatic disease.

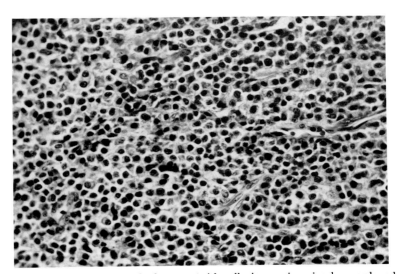

FIG. 1. Uniform mass of plasmacytoid cells in varying size has replaced and distorted a lymph node (H & E 125×).

Malignant Lymphoma, Immunoblastic Sarcoma, B Cell Type, Mediastinum

Clinical History

This 18-year-old Caucasian female was seen for shortness of breath and weakness of four months duration. Chest radiograph demonstrated a poorly defined mass approximately 12 cm in diameter in the anterior mediastinum. Laboratory data included a hemoglobin of 13.4 gm%, WBC of 11,900 with differential of 62 segs, 11 bands, 6 eosinophils, 1 basophil, 7 lymphs and 13 monocytes. At mediastinoscopy, no involved lymph nodes were noted and a small amount of tumor was visualized. Subsequently, a thoracotomy was performed with removal of a nonencapsulated mediastinal mass which was adherent to the major vessels and had to be dissected from the pericardial sac.

Gross Pathology

The specimen weighed 325 gm and measured 14 X 11 X 4 cm. It was roughly triangular, moderately firm rubbery tissue which on cut surface was pink-tan to light red. Some areas were softened with zones of light red-gray discoloration suggesting degenerative change.

Microscopic Findings

The process consisted of a diffuse cellular proliferation without evidence of lymph node or thymic architecture. There were a few areas of fibrosis, but essentially no well-defined collagen bands. The cellular proliferation was moderately variable in size and amount of cytoplasm. The cytoplasm was pale, acidophilic and in areas was prominent in amount, but often limited or even unimpressive. The nuclei were round to oval, have finely dispersed chromatin with several small- to medium-sized nucleoli, often situated in an irregular fashion on the nuclear membrane. Mitoses were infrequent. Plasmacytoid character of the cells in the form of deeply amphophilic cytoplasm or definitely eccentric nuclei were not apparent. The methyl green pyronine stain failed to show a dramatic pyroninophilia, but in this case it is possible that delayed penetration of the fixative prevented staining.

Special Studies

The results of surface marker studies provide conclusive evidence of the B cell nature of this lymphoma. The immunologic surface marker studies reveal 83% of the cells had IgG on their surfaces without any other heavy chains and only 87% of the cells had Ig kappa and none marked with Ig lambda. Thus, the surface immunoglobulin was monoclonal type. None of the cells marked as E rosettes, EAC, or EA rosettes. The cytochemistry studies failed to reveal any cells stained with the nonspecific esterase (histiocytes marker).

Histologic Differential Diagnosis

The differential diagnosis is primarily concerned with a lymphoma of a large cell type or the heterogenous histiocytic type of Rappaport which includes five cell types. In this patient, the large cleaved follicular center cell lymphoma and the true histiocytic as exemplified by Case 18 and the T cell immunoblastic sarcoma can be readily differentiated by the criteria outlined in Case 21. The principal problem is the differentiation between the large noncleaved FCC and the immunoblastic sarcoma of B cell types. Since this case lacks both plasmacytoid feature of the usual IBS and the follicular structures or small cleaved cells as noted in follicular center cell lymphoma, classification is more difficult. On the basis of the prominent nucleoli and cytoplasm, this tumor fits best as immunoblastic sarcoma, although admittedly the process is borderline between IBS and FCC lymphoma. The distinction appears important since our preliminary kinetic studies suggest IBS is much more erratic in ploidy than the large noncleaved FCC. This nuclear feature may be highly significant in predicting the response to therapy. The histologic differential diagnosis is listed in Table 1.

Table 1. Differential Diagnosis

1. Large cleaved FCC lymphoma
2. Histiocytic lymphoma (Rappaport)
3. Immunoblastic sarcoma, T cell type
4. Large noncleaved FCC lymphoma
5. Immunoblastic sarcoma B cell type

Clinical Staging

Lymphangiographic studies failed to reveal any evidence of retroperitoneal involvement and the liver and spleen were normal size by scan. There was no evidence of bone marrow involvement and the clinical stage is I.

Clinical Correlation and Follow-up

This case is a most interesting and challenging diagnostic problem both clinically and morphologically. Clinically, the presentation is unusual because this is a B cell lymphoma occurring as a mediastinal mass in a teenager. The most common mediastinal lymphoma in this age group is the convoluted lymphocytic type which is T cell origin. Furthermore, the B cell lymphomas in children and teenagers are predominately small noncleaved FCC types (the Burkitt-like lymphomas) and have a predominately abdominal (gastrointestinal) presentation. The limited extent of the disease and presentation as clinical stage I is also unusual for this high turnover rate type of proliferation. In our recent clinical pathologic correlation study of 33 cases of IBS the group of cases with clinical stage I or II, without symptoms, or lymphocytopenia had prolonged median survival and the possibility of cure, while the number of cases with disseminated disease as stage III or IV, systemic symptoms and at times lymphocytopenia had a median survival of four months. It appears that IBS when widespread and symptomatic is a rapidly progressive process that poorly responds to therapy, but there is a small proportion of the patients that may still be effectively treated and possibly controlled if recognized at an early stage.

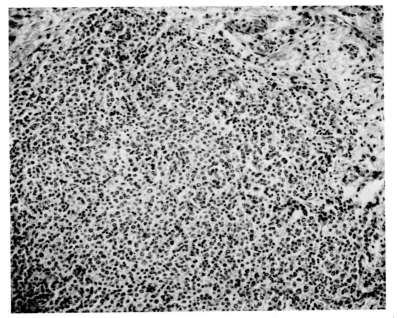

FIG. 1. Diffuse proliferation with no evidence of nodal or thymic architecture in which the cells are fairly uniform and moderate size (H & E 50×).

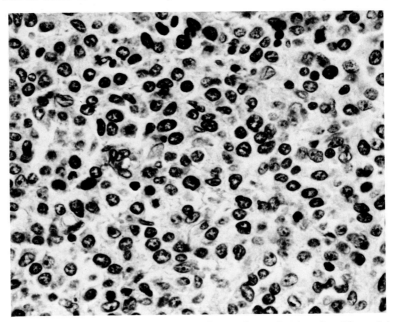

FIG. 2. Cells have moderate amount of cytoplasm that is pale with nuclei that are round to oval with occasional nucleoli. Plasmacytoid features are noted in many cells (H & E 500×).

Malignant Lymphoma, Immunoblastic Sarcoma, Probably B Cell, Cerebrum

Clinical History

This 64-year-old Mexican-American female was admitted September 24, 1975, with an eight-week history of increasing weakness, headache and difficulty in swallowing. For two years she experienced progressive memory loss, disorientation and bizarre behavior. Previously in April 1973 she noted right homonymous hemianopsia, early papillaedema, increased muscle tone, slight nuchal rigidity and bilateral Babinski signs. At that time, echoencephalogram revealed a 4 mm right to left shift and a right carotid angiogram showed an avascular right frontal parietal mass. The brain scan showed an abnormal uptake in several areas. She was treated with steroids and radiation of 3000 rads. She improved clinically and subsequently the scan showed no areas of abnormal uptake.

September 1975 she had early papillaedema, left homonymous hemianopsia, cogwheel rigidity, decreased strength on the right and bilateral Babinski signs. A brain scan showed increased uptake on the left frontal parietal area. A right carotid angiogram revealed a left parasagittal cerebral filling defect. A tumor was suspected and she was discharged to a nursing home and died January 13, 1976. Tissue was obtained from the autopsy for the conference.

Gross Pathology

Coronal sections of the cerebrum showed a well-circumscribed white tumor measuring 2.0 × 1.5 cm and located on the superior, anterior left frontal lobe extending into the subarachnoid space. Posteriorly, the left frontal mass on cut section measured 3 × 2 cm. In the right frontal lobe

there was another well-circumscribed mass measuring 6 × 6 ×
5 cm and lying 4 cm lateral to the midline. A distinct third
mass measuring 4 × 3 cm was noted in the body of the
corpus callosum. Several other well-circumscribed masses were
noted in the globus pallidus and left thalamus. The autopsy
cause of death was bronchopneumonia. Search of the lymph
nodes at autopsy showed none to be enlarged or contain
apparent tumor. The spleen weight was 110 gm and no tumor
nodules were noted. A meningioma of the right frontal aspect
of the dura measuring 0.5 cm in diameter was an incidental
finding.

Microscopic Findings

This specimen was post therapy and some cytologic distor-
tion and necrosis may be partially attributable to therapy.
The massive infiltrate of the cerebral cortex was fairly well
demarcated at one margin of the specimen. Within the specimen there were areas of obvious necrosis, technical artifacts
and small areas of hemorrhage. The cellular infiltration
extended up to the left meninges and cells were scattered
within the subarachnoid space. The finding had potential
significance because lymphoma cells may be obtained in the
spinal fluid and concentrated by cytocentrifuge technique,
characterized with immunologic surface marker studies and
cytochemical procedures, even though the number of cells
within the CSF is limited. Higher magnification demonstrated
the cells were loosely arranged and noncohesive. The cells
were large and most were two to five times the size of small
lymphocytic nuclei. Usually a prominent amount of acidophilic staining cytoplasm with fairly demarcated cellular
borders was noted. The nuclei varied remarkably in size and
configuration in the more superficial and better preserved
portions of the specimen. A component of the population is
round to oval and the cells bear a definite resemblance to
transformed lymphocytes. Nucleoli were identified but largely
obscured. The nuclear chromatin was finely depressed, mitotic
figures were prominent and the cells did not demonstrate a
recognizable plasmacytoid character.

Special Studies

The immunoperoxidase stains for cytoplasmic immuno-globulin were extremely helpful. Monoclonal cytoplasmic immunoglobulin of IgG kappa type was found, indicating B cell origin.

Histologic Differential Diagnosis

When several sections were examined, no other tumor was considered. The degree of pleomorphism excludes oligoden-droglioma. Occasionally, germinoma occurs in the pineal area, but is not as pleomorphic as this tumor. Furthermore, ger-minoma is not multicentric with the CNS as noted in this patient.

Precise classification within the large cell lymphomas is somewhat difficult if severe alterations resulting from post-mortem changes and therapy are present. The marked ir-regularity in nuclear configuration suggests a large cleaved FCC lymphoma, but we believe this cellular irregularity is primarily artifactual. The numerous mitoses support a trans-formed lymphocyte proliferation that is irregular in configura-tion. The distinction between a large noncleaved FCC and IBS of B cell types is extremely difficult if not impossible in the postmortem and post therapy state. The diagnosis of IBS is principally based on the prominence of immunoglobulin found in the immunoperoxidase stains and the demonstration of IgG kappa.

Clinical Staging

Primary CNS lymphoma are nearly always restricted to the CNS and staging is not usually performed.

Clinical Correlation and Follow-up

In the past few years it has become apparent that lym-phomatous involvement of the central nervous system is not uncommon in systemic lymphoma. It is a frequent complica-tion of the lymphoma-leukemia process of children, specific-ally the convoluted T cell type. In adults, CNS involvement also occurs as a late complication of lymphomas, usually classified as histiocytic lymphoma. Approximately 30% of the patients in the series of 52 reported by Bunn et al developed CNS complications that commonly were leptomeningeal [1]. The spread of lymphoma into CNS is distinctive. The leukemic type involvement which is principally of T cell type essentially is superficial and meningeal but may extend into the underlying cortex and perivascular locations. With a greater effectiveness of combination chemotherapy in systemic lymphoma and with patients living longer, it seems likely that there will be an increased frequency of CNS involvement and pathologists will be called upon to establish a diagnosis of lymphomas on specimens of various types. Of particular importance will be the recognition of the cytologic types of malignant lymphoma in concentrated specimens of the spinal fluid where small numbers of cells may be available. In the report of Bunn et al the diagnosis was established in all ten by spinal fluid examination. The initial manifestation of lymphoma of the CNS may first be apparent as opacities of the vitreous [2].

The clinical presentation of a primary CNS lymphoma is not distinctive from other brain tumors. However, it is now also acknowledged that lymphomas may arise in and be limited to the central nervous system [3,4] and can be readily distinguished from the primary glial tumors. Special studies were useful, and 19 of 24 patients examined showed staining for immunoglobulin (immunoperoxidase), although 13 cases had sufficient staining to allow interpretation. Interestingly, some astrocytes around the tumor also stained for immunoglobulin although this staining was polyclonal [4].

References

1. Bunn, P.A., Schein, P.S., Banks, P.M.: Central nervous system complications in patients with diffuse histiocytic and undifferentiated lymphoma; Leukemia revisited. Blood 47:3-10, 1976.
2. Minckler, D.S., Font, R.L. and Zimmerman, L.E.: Uveitis and reticulum cell sarcoma of brain with bilateral neoplastic seeding of vitreous without retinal or uveal involvement. Am. J. Ophthalmol. 80:433-439, 1975.

3. Henry, J.M., Heffner, R.R., Dillar, S.H. et al: Primary malignant lymphoma of the central nervous system. Cancer 34:1293-1302, 1974.
4. Taylor, C.R., Russell, R., Lukes, R.J. and Davis, R.L.: An immuno-histological study of immunoglobulin content of primary central nervous system lymphomas. Cancer 41:2197-2205, 1978.

III
T Cell Lesions

Convoluted Lymphocytic Lymphoma-Leukemia (T Cell), Mediastinum

Clinical History

This 8-year-old Mexican-American male was in good health until one week prior to admission, when he returned from school with a stomach ache. Five days prior to admission he noted gum bleeding and had difficulty speaking. He also vomited once a day and noted little "speckles" over his body. On admission he could not work or move his left arm and initially lost consciousness. On physical examination, the child was comatose with labored respiration and vomiting. The right pupil was fixed and dilated, whereas the left pupil was responsive. Several small lymph nodes were palpated in the anterior cervical and posterior cervical areas. The lungs had bilateral rales, the liver was 14 cm in length by percussion and the spleen was palpated 3 cm below the costal margin. Numerous shoddy lymph nodes were palpated in the groin. Shortly after admission, both pupils became fixed and dilated and hemorrhages were noted on fundoscopic examination. The WBC was 500,000 cells/mm^3 and most of these cells were reported as lymphoblasts. A bone marrow aspirate revealed predominantly blasts. The child died within 24 hours of admission.

Gross Pathology

An autopsy revealed a mediastinal large firm, yellow-white nodular mass measuring 18 × 14 cm and weighing 250 gm. The mass was removed from the thymic area and was attached to the anterior pericardium. Surrounding lymph nodes were enlarged, irregular and firm, measuring up to 3.5 × 2.0 cm. In the central portion, a 2.5 × 1.5 cm cavity with a mildly trabecular inner surface was noted. The liver weight was 1400 gm and the

95

spleen weight was 350 gm. A large right intracerebral hemorrhage with rupture of the cerebrum was noted and there was blood in subarachnoid space. There was some cerebellar herniation, more marked on the right than on the left.

Microscopic Findings

The sections provided for study are from the mediastinal mass and they exhibit a diffuse infiltrative process without any evidence of architectural features. No remnants of thymus are found. The cellular proliferation exhibits a range in cell size from that of a small lymphocyte nucleus to 3 to 4 lymphocyte nuclear diameters. The cells have scanty or inapparent cytoplasm and are noncohesive. Often the cells are loosely arranged and fairly widely separated. This latter feature may be the result of postmortem changes. The nuclear configuration is variable but often irregular, and on close inspection the nuclei have a somewhat convoluted appearance with nodular-like projections or linear subdivisions. This latter feature varies in degree and often must be closely searched for to be discerned. In areas the nuclear linear subdivisions are numerous though fine and are definitely reminiscent of the lateral surface of the cerebral cortex. In a few areas the nuclei of the larger cells are subdivided and even appear lobated. The nuclear chromatin is finely dispersed, but can readily be obscured in somewhat overstained sections. Mitotic figures are numerous and in postmortem sections often are much less apparent.

Special Studies

Unfortunately no multiparameter studies were performed on this case. The patient was admitted on Saturday night and died within 24 hours. In such patients with circulating abnormal cells, the studies may be accomplished by collecting and refrigerating cells and preparing multiple smears for cytochemical procedures. We have been able to accomplish immunologic surface markers with specimens held overnight and, on a few occasions, as long as 48 hours later. In our series of over 30 cases of convoluted lymphocytic lymphoma-leukemia, the convoluted lymphocytes form E rosettes, but the frequency is extremely variable with the numbers ranging from 5% to 90%.

The significance of this wide range is uncertain, but there appears to be a relationship between the frequency of E rosettes and the degree of convolutions. In a number of cases EAC rosettes have also been demonstrated usually in those cases with high numbers of E rosettes. It now appears that the convoluted 'T' cell has a C_3 receptor and Stein et al have interpreted this as evidence of the pre-T cell nature of the convoluted T cell since the thymic cells of human fetuses before 14 months possess a C_3 receptor [1]. The surface immunoglobulin usually is extremely low and both Stein et al and Catovsky have demonstrated consistent acid phosphatase positivity with the occurrence of large positive globules in the vicinity of the Golgi apparatus. They believe that this is a reliable marker for the convoluted T cell and T cell ALL. There are technical problems, however, that in our view make this difficult to reproduce. Ideally, the smears or touch imprints should be air-dried and according to Lennert (personal communication) held for at least 24 hours before performing the procedure or the enzyme does not appear to be active. This observation suggests the conversion from pro-enzyme to an active state. From our experience with a large series of cases, it appears that the results of the surface marker studies are highly predictive from the morphologic features and the acid phosphatase positivity may be effective if the material is collected and prepared and applied precisely. It is acknowledged that all childhood cases with mediastinal masses may not be convoluted, as pointed out by Nathwani et al [2]. In one of our case series, four of the patients presented with small noncleaved FCC type diffuse, and it is suspected that occasional cases may be of the U cell type. In the immediate future it is essential that as many cases as possible with mediastinal masses be characterized by multiparameter studies to determine the discriminating character of the morphologic features.

Histologic Differential Diagnosis

There are four conditions principally in the differential diagnosis and are listed as follows:
1. Acute lymphocytic leukemia
2. Burkitt and Burkitt-like lymphomas
    (small noncleaved FCC)

3. Primitive infiltrative tumors
4. Thymoma

Acute lymphocytic leukemia of childhood is now acknowledged to be a heterogeneous group of disorders that includes the T cell type which interrelates with the convoluted lymphocytic lymphoma, the B cell type, which is a small noncleaved FCC type, and the nonmarking or so-called null cell type. In excellent histologic sections the distinction between these three subtypes presently included in ALL can be readily distinguished, but in thick sections of improperly fixed tissue the differential diagnosis may be difficult. Using a methyl green pyronine stain to demonstrate the cytoplasm, the distinction can be greatly simplified. The B cell type has prominent pyroninophilic cytoplasm with cohesive cellular borders; whereas the convoluted T cell has scanty or almost inapparent pyroninophilic cytoplasm; while the null cell has a rather narrow rim of pyroninophilic cytoplasm and small nucleoli. All three cytologic types have primitive-appearing nuclei, but the convoluted nucleus has distinctive linear subdivisions that produce the convoluted appearance. In smears and touch imprints of biopsy material all three cell types have basophilic cytoplasm with the convoluted lymphocyte having limited amount of cytoplasm, the small noncleaved the most abundant, and it is commonly vacuolated while the null cell is intermediate.

The Burkitt and Burkitt-like lymphoma are small noncleaved FCC lymphoma and are interrelated with the B cell leukemia described above. The third consideration, primitive tumors of various types, may present considerable difficulty in diagnosis depending upon the site of involvement and especially in childhood. In these essentially primordial tumors excellently prepared sections are essential. It is to be remembered that the convoluted T cell may present as infiltrative masses in many sites and therefore must be included in the differential diagnosis of all primitive tumors. The fourth consideration in the differential diagnosis, thymoma, is important because in a sense the convoluted T cell, particularly presenting as a mediastinal mass, is a malignant thymoma. It should be emphasized, however, that we are uncertain at the present time whether the process develops in the thymus or is infiltrated from a pre-T cell that migrates from another source such as the bone marrow.

This consideration is supported by the recent observation that the convoluted T cell with C_3 receptor is similar to the human fetal thymic cell prior to 14 weeks gestation. On this basis the convoluted T cell has been thought to be a pre-T cell. Thymomas of lymphocytic type, however, are composed of small T lymphocytes and can be readily distinguished from the convoluted T cell.

Clinical Correlation and Follow-up

In this case the presentation was unusual with central nervous system symptoms and hemorrhage with bleeding gums and petechiae. There was respiratory obstruction due to the mass, vomiting and eventually coma. The cerebrum did show leukemic infiltration.

The clinical presentation in the convoluted T cell type commonly is associated with a mediastinal mass. At times the mediastinal mass is a dramatic component and is associated with respiratory obstruction. At times the respiratory obstruction may present problems in administering anesthesia or even achieving biopsy. Respiratory obstruction may be so extreme that it may be life-threatening. Rapid death is common and five of our cases died on the day of admission, two of which occurred during the induction of anesthesia. Interpretation of this process as lymphomatous or acute lymphocytic leukemia is dependent upon the presentation. In the past, if features of acute leukemia were encountered, such as petechiae and purpura or leukemia peripheral blood, the process has been considered an acute lymphocytic leukemia, even though a mediastinal mass was present. This condition has appeared in the literature for a number of years as ALL with mediastinal mass. If an identical mediastinal mass was present without obvious leukemia, then the process was interpreted as a lymphoma, even though the cellular proliferation was identical. In our view the process is a lymphoma-leukemia with variations in the presentation depending upon the moment of initial observation of the patient and some variation in the extramarrow presentations [3]. The variations in the clinical presentation of our initial report of the convoluted T cell is recorded in Table 1. Twenty patients (74%) were discovered to have a mediastinal mass, 17 of the 27 had lymphadenopathy principally in the cervical and supraclavicular regions [4].

Leukemic peripheral blood or marrow was discovered at the time of initial observation in 11 of the 27 cases. Nine subsequently became leukemia; seven either at the time of last follow-up or at death had no marrow or peripheral blood involvement. The median survival was ten months and only one patient had survived beyond two years. The findings in the second series of cases, a study of lymphomas of the Childrens Hospital of Los Angeles, which included 56 cases of the convoluted T cell, presented with very similar clinical features with 52% of the cases having a mediastinal mass [5]. The median survival in this larger group is also ten months.

Following therapy of various types, disease commonly relapses within six months commonly in the marrow and often in the central nervous system. In the cases we have observed since completion of our two case series mentioned above, essentially all of the cases have relapsed in six months and all had involvement of the central nervous system.

The response to therapy is commonly dramatic but the relapse within three to six months in almost all cases is equally dramatic, and induction of remission almost never occurs. Mediastinal masses rapidly disappear with radiation therapy or the usual acute chemotherapy for ALL. Recently, it has been demonstrated by Ohnuma et al that the cells of T cell ALL are L-asparagine dependent which accounts for the occasional dramatic responses of ALL to L-asparaginase [6]. In the past it has been generally acknowledged that therapy for lymphomas of childhood has been totally ineffective essentially with all cases dying within a year. Recently, Wollner et al demonstrated a dramatic change in the response with a complicated nine agent therapeutic regimen, the so-called L-2 approach, which incidentally includes L-asparaginase [7]. The dramatic difference in reported survival which is complete departure of all previous

Table 1. Clinical Features of Convoluted Lymphocytic Lymphoma

Mediastinal mass	20/27
Respiratory obstruction	6/20
Lymphadenopathy without mediastinal mass	6/27
Leukemia at diagnosis	11/27
Leukemia after diagnosis	10/16

reports raises an issue regarding the cytologic types within the treated group and emphasizes the need in the future for the use of multiparameter techniques to insure the comparability of case populations in protocol studies. It is also interesting that in this study of 35 cases, six were interpreted as nodular lymphoma poorly differentiated lymphocytic type of Rappaport, an almost nonexistent cytologic type in our experience in childhood. In my experience through the years and in our recent study of a 25-year period of the Childrens Hospital of Los Angeles population, all of the childhood cases presented with a diffuse histologic pattern and only one case contained one microscopic field with a nodular (follicular) pattern.

In summary, the multiparameter approach will allow better separation of these childhood diseases. The prognostic importance and therapeutic value of this classification are under review and preliminary results have been published [3].

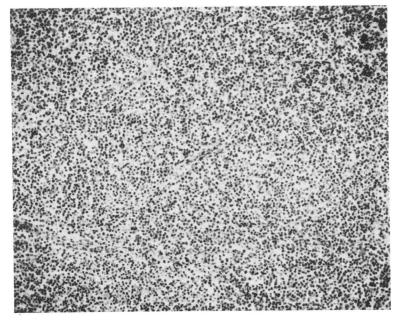

FIG. 1. Diffuse noncohesive cellular proliferation of primitive-appearing cells (H & E 50×).

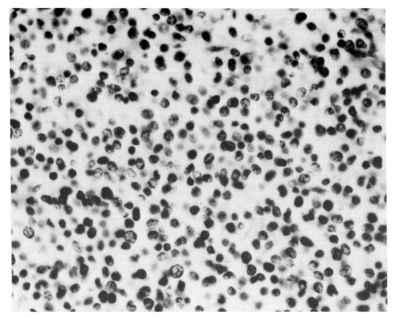

FIG. 2. Proliferation exhibits a range in cell size from one to four lymphocytic nuclear diameters. The larger cells have finely dispersed chromatin and a few have fine linear subdivisions. On close inspection, occasional cells have irregular nuclear margins (H & E 500×).

References

1. Stein, H., Petersen, N., Gaedicke, et al: Lymphoblastic lymphoma of convoluted or acid phosphatase type — A tumor of T precursor cells. Int. J. Cancer 17:292-295, 1976.
2. Nathwani, B.N., Kim, H. and Rappaport, H.: Malignant lymphoma, lymphoblastic. Cancer 38:964-983, 1976.
3. Williams, H.A., Taylor, C.R., Higgins, G.R. et al: Childhood lymphoma-leukemia. I. Correlation of morphology and immunological studies. Cancer 42:171-181, 1978.
4. Barcos, M.P. and Lukes, R.J.: Malignant lymphoma of convoluted lymphocytes: A new entity of possible T-Cell type. In Sinks, L.F. and Godden, J.O. (eds.): Conflicts in Childhood Cancer. An Evaluation of Current Management. New York:Alan R. Liss, Inc., 1975, Vol. 4, pp. 147-178.
5. Schneider, B.K., Higgins, G.R., Swanson, V. et al: Malignant lymphomas in childhood. Blood 46:1015, 1975.
6. Ohnuma, T., Orlowski, M., Minowada, J. et al: Differences in amino acid metabolism of human T- and B-cells in culture. Proceedings XVI

International Congress of Hematology. Kyoto, Japan, September 1976, p. 220.

7. Wollner, N., Lieberman, P., Exelby, P. et al: Non-Hodgkin's lymphoma in children: Results of treatment with LSA_2-L_2 protocol. J. Cancer 31:337-342, 1975.

Malignant Lymphoma, Mycosis Fungoides (T Cell), Skin and Axillary Lymph Node

Clinical History

This 48-year-old black female was admitted for evaluation of dry pruritic skin lesions of the upper extremities and trunk which have been present for three years. One year previously, similar skin lesions were noted on the face. These multiple lesions were nodular, slightly violaceous with superficial scaling and on the face were up to 3.5 cm in diameter. The arms and trunk were covered with small 1 mm diameter papules. Several small lymph nodes 1 to 2 cm in diameter were palpated in the right submental area, left anterior cervical area and left axilla. Laboratory data included a hemoglobin of 14 gm%, WBC of 8800 with a normal differential count. A skin biopsy and lymph node biopsy were obtained.

Microscopic Findings

In the skin biopsy there is a heavy abnormal lymphocytic infiltration in the mid and deep portions of the dermis that concentrates in a somewhat nodular fashion about the epidermal appendages and rete pegs. The most superficial portion of the dermis, the so-called Grenz zone, is lightly infiltrated. The overlying epidermis is only slightly thickened. There is no evidence of a psoriaform type of epidermal proliferation. At intermediate magnification it is apparent that the cellular infiltrate is intimately associated with the appendages and deeper portions of the rete pegs with loss of demarcation and extension of the infiltrate into the epidermis. Collections of the abnormal cells are found in forming typical Pautrier's abscesses. The cellular proliferation within the dermis is extremely abnormal, primitive appearing and essentially monomorphous. Mitotic figures are frequent. These cells vary moderately in size and configuration, have finely dispersed nuclear chromatin, usually a medium-size basophilic nucleolus and a moderate amount of cytoplasm with indistinct cellular borders. The nuclear margins at times are irregular. The linear subdivisions resembling the cerebriform cells of Sezary's syndrome are not readily discernible, though irregular projections from the nuclear membrane at times are apparent. Cells have only lightly pyroninophilic cytoplasm.

The lymph node is altered partially by an abnormal cellular infiltration of the paracortical area leaving circumscribed and uninvolved reactive follicles with their lymphocytic mantles. The abnormal cellular infiltration is essentially similar to that described above in the dermis, with the exception that the nuclear configuration in areas is more irregular.

Special Studies

The functional studies are consistent with a lymph node with reactive follicles because there is polyclonal marking. However, cytocentrifuge studies indicated the lymphomatous cells formed E rosettes. This important observation emphasizes what has been appreciated in our study of T cell lymphoma. Namely, that review of the functional studies of T cell lesions requires cytocentrifuge study to verify that the abnormal cell is forming E rosettes.

Electron microscopy of the lymphomatous areas revealed cells with the typical cerebriform nuclei of the Sezary cell.

	E	EAC	EA	PV	M	G	A	D	κ	λ
Peripheral blood	76	6	0	29	18	21	1	8	31	16
Lymph node	47	2	0	32	16	7	3	14	22	17

Histologic Differential Diagnosis

The principal problem of differential diagnosis involves three groups of lesions: (1) those lesions with psoriaform epidermal proliferation with heavy mixed dermal infiltration, (2) dissemination of generalized lymphoma with cutaneous tumor nodules, particularly extending to the superficial dermis and (3) the pseudolymphomas of the skin. With experience, pseudolymphomas can be readily distinguished and, in a sense, are not part of the differential diagnosis of this case.

A number of lesions have prominent psoriaform epidermal proliferations with varying degrees of cellular infiltration. At times the infiltration may be heavy and extend through the Grenz zone. On occasion epidermal infiltrations resembling Pautrier's abscesses are noted. For the diagnosis of mycosis fungoides on a purely morphologic basis, a heavy infiltrate in the plaque phase broadly extending through the superficial Grenz zone is required. It is of mixed composition in this phase and the cellular infiltrate includes a full range of cells with plasma cells, transformed lymphocytes or immunoblasts, eosinophils and histiocytes. Sezary cells with their characteristic cerebriform nuclei may be identified on electron microscopy, but it would be extremely difficult to identify these cells in H & E stained histologic sections. Thus, the distinguishing features of mycosis fungoides are primarily the psoriaform character of the epidermal proliferation, the distribution of the infiltrate extending throughout the mid and superficial dermis and its mixed composition in the plaque phase. Ideally, characterization of the cellular infiltration should be a requirement, but often the cellular details are greatly distorted, particularly in the small punch biopsies, and it is difficult to put the needed reliance on this component.

Disseminated malignant lymphoma involving the skin, on the other hand, depends upon identification of specific cytologic types and may be impossible on small distorted or punch biopsies. Through the years, having the opportunity to study large numbers of lymphoid lesions of the skin and possible lymphomas, we have found an approach which has effectively handled such problems. In patients with previously diagnosed malignant lymphoma who develop tumor lymphoid nodules in the skin, the question arises: Does the cutaneous nodule sufficiently resemble pretherapy diagnostic lymph node biopsy, or does it represent a more aggressive expression of the process? Usually these two expressions can be reconciled if the skin biopsy is processed properly. On the other hand, in patients presenting with tumor nodules in the skin without a previous diagnosis of lymphoma on a lymph node biopsy, we have insisted on a thorough search for evidence of lymphomatous involvement outside of the skin even if the lymphoma cytologically fulfills the criteria for malignant lymphoma. From our experience, this has proven to be very reliable in patients with biopsies fulfilling the cytologic criteria since they have had disease elsewhere and are stage IV disease that was usually rapidly progressive. When the cytologic feature did not fulfill the criteria of malignant lymphoma, no lymphoma has been found elsewhere. The third area of differential diagnosis, the pseudolymphoma of the skin, involves a wide variety of lesions that are most frequently and predominantly lymphocytic. These lesions occur principally in three forms: (1) perivascular and periepidicular nodules, (2) diffuse dermal infiltrates and (3) large single nodules which may present as tumor nodules that extend through the dermis. The cellular proliferation though predominantly lymphocytic commonly is associated with plasma cells, a small number of immunoblasts and a reactive mesenchymal or histiocytic component. At times small follicles with reaction centers may be found. In rare instances large follicles with reaction centers have been encountered. In conjunction with Dr. Paul Hirsch, a dermatopathologist, criteria for differentiating these processes from malignant lymphoma were presented [1]. Recognition of pseudolymphomatous reactions is not based upon extent of involvement, but on the mixed cellular composition with its reactive components of histiocytes, plasma cells and immunoblasts and often proliferating vessels. The epidermis is essentially uninvolved or may be thin over the nodular proliferations.

Staging

Through the decades mycosis fungoides was considered essentially to be limited to the skin with few exceptions. Recent studies using exploratory laparotomies and staging of patients with mycosis fungoides have demonstrated a surprisingly high frequency of not only lymph node involvement, but dissemination to spleen and abdominal lymph nodes [2].

Clinical Correlations and Follow-up

This patient had good response to chemotherapy but experienced relapse with widespread cutaneous lesions and visceral lesions. She died of sepsis 20 months after diagnosis.

The clinical presentation with a leonine facies (lionlike) is unusual, but has been described. The predominant involvement of the skin by lymphoma as the initial observation is also uncommon, but has been described under the term mycosis fungoides d'emblee, a term used for the type of lymphoma presenting initially in the tumor stage. This patient had lymph node involvement at the time of initial observation.

Mycosis fungoides and Sezary's syndrome are now both accepted as T cell processes. Through the years we have been reluctant to include mycosis fungoides in the malignant lymphomas because of its principal involvement of the skin. With our present knowledge of the T cell nature of both mycosis fungoides and Sezary's syndrome it appears that these processes should be included in malignant lymphomas as a T cell subtype with this type of lymphoma selectively either arising in the skin or principally involving the skin, and the T cell portions of lymph node and spleen. The relationship between mycosis fungoides and Sezary's syndrome has been debated, but Lutzner recently has indicated that he believes that Sezary's syndrome is a leukemic expression of mycosis fungoides [3]. It would seem reasonable to place mycosis fungoides and Sezary's in the same group within the T cell lymphomas: Sezary's being the leukemic expression and mycosis fungoides the disorder with plaque and tumor phases, though admittedly we are uncertain what cytologic characteristics determine these expressions.

The functional behavior of the cerebriform cell of mycosis fungoides and Sezary's syndrome has been unknown. Recently, Broder et al presented evidence indicating that the Sezary cell had the functional characteristics of helper T cells and participated in this manner in immunologic reaction, aiding in B cells in the production of immunoglobulin and antibodies [4]. Whether mycosis fungoides cells function in a similar fashion is unknown.

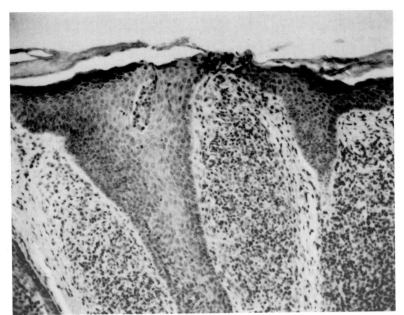

FIG. 1. Skin biopsy with intense cellular proliferation in the superficial dermis. There is intimate proximity to the overlying and adjacent epithelium with extension of small numbers of cells into the epithelium (H & E 50×).

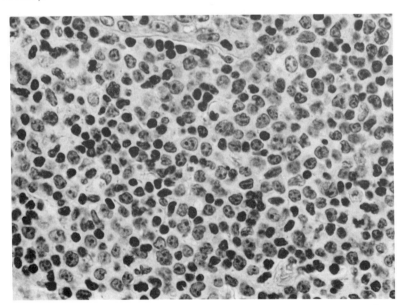

FIG. 2. Skin biopsy: cellular proliferation within the dermis varies from small cells with irregular nuclei to large mononuclear cells with the features of transformed nuclei. These latter cells have finely dispersed chromatin, one to three small nucleoli and indistinct cytoplasmic borders (H & E 500×).

References

1. Hirsch, P. and Lukes, R.J.: Cutaneous Lymphoid Proliferations I. How does the skin react. II. Specific Cutaneous Lymphoid Reactions. III. Reactive Cutaneous Pseudolymphoma. Proc. Pac. Derm. Assoc. Inc., 1965, pp 35-41.
2. Rappaport, H. and Thomas, L.B.: Mycosis fungoides: The pathology of extracutaneous involvement. Cancer 34:1198-1229, 1974.
3. Lutzner, M., Edelson, R., Schein, P. et al: Cutaneous T-cell lymphomas: The Sezary syndrome, mycosis fungoides and related disorders. Ann. Intern. Med. 83:534-552, 1975.
4. Broder, S., Edelson, R.L., Lutzner, M.A. et al: The Sezary syndrome: A malignant proliferation of helper T cells. J. Clin. Invest. 58:1297-1306, 1976.

IV
Histiocytic Lesions

Malignant Histiocytosis, Axillary Lymph Node

Clinical History

This 25-year-old black male was admitted in January 1969 for migratory myalgia and temperature of 105 to 106°F. He was previously hospitalized for fever, chills, sore throat and cough at which time small cervical and supraclavicular lymph nodes were palpated. Subsequently, multiple neurologic, cardiac, respiratory, renal and hepatic manifestations were observed, but these complaints improved spontaneously. On the current admission, the temperature was 102°F. A few small cervical and submandibular lymph nodes were palpated and there was left quadraceps weakness and tenderness. A lymphangiogram was abnormal and an axillary lymph node was biopsied.

Gross Pathology

The specimen consisted of fragments measuring 4 × 2.5 × 0.7 cm. Portions were hemorrhagic and fibrofatty tissue. One area was yellow-white semi-soft, homogenous tissue measuring 0.7 cm in diameter.

Microscopic Findings

The histologic material is not ideal because of technical inadequacies of the original fixation and processing, but the specimen represents the pretherapy biopsy of a typical example of this extraordinary disorder. There is artifactual disruption and cracking of the specimen and drying of portions of the specimens in the periphery that obscures the cytologic detail. Nevertheless, the typical features can be discerned in the more ideal portions of the specimens. The lymph node is involved in a most unusual irregular fashion. Three essential diagnostic features are found involving the node in a limited fashion. First, the presence of neoplastic-appearing histiocytes are scattered individually and in clusters in sinusoids. These cells are large with abundant cytoplasm and are known as the prohistiocyte. Second, large pleomorphic and even bizarre lobated and multinucleated cells known as the pleomorphic histiocytes are present. Third, large benign-appearing histiocytes with abundant acidophilic cytoplasm typically containing erythrocytes known as the erythrophagocyte are noted. In this case, the prohistiocytes are observed in varying number scattered individually within the node in sinusoids and in the interfollicular tissue. They are among the normal lymphoid tissue in areas, occur in high concentrations and may dominate the sinusoidal population. Nowhere do they diffusely involve and replace the node. There is no infiltration of the capsule. On high magnification the mononuclear or prohistiocytic forms range from 5 to 7 lymphocyte nuclear diameters, have round to oval nuclei and finely dispersed chromatin with usually one medium size nucleolus. The cytoplasm is usually moderate in amount and appears densely amphophilic. The pleomorphic form has two or more often separate nuclei with the same appearance with more abundant cytoplasm. They are in the range of megakaryocytes in size. The cytoplasm of both the mononuclear and pleomorphic cells is intensely pyroninophilic. The unusual feature of the initial biopsy was the lack of prominent benign-appearing phagocytes with erythrophagocytosis. In a comparison study of the postmortem cellular proliferation of lymph nodes, the cytologic details are more ideally portrayed since the material was carefully collected. Erythrophagocytosis is dramatic and benign erythrophagocytes are prominent. There is an increase in the connective tissue in the intersinusoidal or interfollicular tissue, but the tissue was collected at the post therapy state. The cytologic features of the prohistiocytes and pleomorphic histiocytes are essentially similar.

Special Studies

The study in this case was limited to histologic methods, since this was encountered in 1969, several years before the multiparameter technique program was instituted.

Histologic Differential Diagnosis

A recognition of this lesion generally is not difficult after one acquires considerable experience, but in general there are two types of processes in lymph nodes which produce difficulty: (1) abnormal cellular proliferations with prominent sinusoidal components and erythrophagocytosis and (2) pleomorphic cellular proliferations associated with lobation and multinucleation, including Hodgkin's disease and immunoblastic sarcoma. The former condition (abnormal immune reaction) is excluded because intermediate expressions of transformed lymphocytes are not recognized in this case. In regard to the second category, needle biopsies of liver, marrow aspirates, smears and particle sections the differential diagnosis may involve pleomorphic cells of various types and conditions associated with erythrophagocytosis. The differential diagnosis is achieved principally on the recognition of the prohistiocyte and the pleomorphic histiocyte and their distinction from metastatic tumors without primary reliance upon the presence of erythrophagocytosis. Thus, they may be supported by cytochemical procedures such as the alpha naphthyl butyrate for histiocytes or the immunoperoxidase stain on paraffin sections for muramidase. When erythrophagocytosis is encountered in sinusoids of lymph nodes, the pathologist must be cautious since this phenomenon occurs in the regional nodes of petechiae and ecchymoses or any hemorrhage, and the critical cells, prohistiocytes and pleomorphic histiocytes must be identified. Thus, cytologic identification under both conditions is of paramount importance. The prohistiocyte is a large cell that resembles somewhat a huge transformed lymphocyte. On less than optimum material, the distinction may be difficult cytologically. Fortunately, immunoblasts are uncommonly found in sinusoids and are usually not multinucleated. The distinction of this disorder from Hodgkin's disease is also assisted by the rarity of Reed-Sternberg cells being found in sinusoids of lymph nodes or hepatic sinusoids. The cytologic distinction therefore on individual cells may be difficult, but the affinity for these malignant histiocytes for sinusoids greatly simplifies the distinction of the differential diagnosis.

Clinical Staging

None performed.

Clinical Correlation and Follow-up

The initial period of hospitalization in the fall of 1968, with fever, chills, sore throat and expressions of a multisystem disease from which the patient spontaneously improved, was extremely puzzling to the clinicians, and it is uncertain whether it relates to the histiocytic medullary reticulosis. The manifestations observed clinically at the time of the second admission in early 1969 with migratory muscle pains, shaking chills with spike fever of 105° to 106°, slight cervical lymphadenopathy, left axillary lymphadenopathy and slight hepatomegaly seemed likely to be expressions of this disorder. At the time of the biopsy of the left axillary lymph node the hemoglobin was 12.6, the hematocrit 39% and WBC count of 8,000. An anemia developed only after the institution of therapy. This case lacks one of the most dramatic clinical expressions, a hemolytic anemia. It was noted that erythrophagocytosis was also essentially absent, though it was prominent at autopsy. Peripheral lymphadenopathy also was not conspicuous and splenomegaly was absent. There was no evidence in the bone marrow to suggest the diagnosis of histiocytic medullary reticulosis. Thus the clinical presentations in both admissions were atypical and jaundice was lacking.

Following the institution of combination chemotherapy with prednisone, nitrogen mustary, methylhydrazine and vincristine, he promptly became afebrile, his appetite improved and he began to gain weight. Following the fourth course of chemotherapy, however, he relapsed with severe anemia and leukopenia and died suddenly six months after diagnosis and approximately ten months after first symptoms.

At autopsy there was 1 liter of clear yellow fluid in the peritoneal cavity. The liver weight was 2280 gm and the spleen weight was 950 gm. Both organs had microscopic deposition of tumor. The lymph nodes were enlarged in all areas and the lungs showed bronchopneumonia. Scattered tumor nodules (0.2 to 2 cm in diameter) were noted in the pericardium, myocardium, ureter, small bowel serosa, pancreas and bone marrow.

Malignant histiocytosis was originally called histiocytic medullary reticulosis and over 100 examples have now been published [1]. Recently, a number of cases have occurred in patients under treatment for acute lymphocytic leukemia [2]. It was suggested that these two diseases may have a common stem cell.

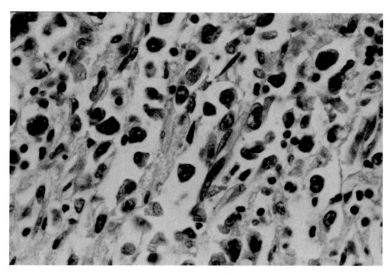

FIG. 1. Malignant histiocytosis: abnormal histiocytes are unattached within small vascular spaces. These cells vary from mononuclear cells with prominent nuclei and moderate amount of cytoplasm to large pleomorphic forms (H & E 500X).

References

1. Warnke, R.A., Kim, H., Dorfman, R.F.: Malignant histiocytosis (histiocytic medullary reticulosis). Cancer 35:215-230, 1975.
2. Karcher, D.S., Head, D.R. and Mullins, J.D.: Malignant histiocytosis occurring in patients with acute lymphocytic leukemia. Cancer 41:1967-1973, 1978.

Malignant Lymphoma, Histiocytic Type, Inguinal Lymph Node

Clinical History

This 18-year-old male was first seen in June 1976 because of anorexia, cough, fever (104°) and night sweats. Chest radiograph showed bilateral hilar adenopathy. An enlarged spleen and normal liver size was reported by scan. Failing to respond to antibiotic therapy, a cervical lymph node was removed. The bone scan was normal; a gallium scan showed increased uptake in the perihilar mediastinal region, more prominent on the right side. Skin tests for tuberculosis and coccidioides immitis were negative. A bone marrow was interpreted as showing no lymphoma. In July 1976, a thoracotomy with lung biopsy and mediastinal node biopsy were performed. Difficulty in histopathologic interpretation led to a subsequent biopsy and functional studies.

Gross Pathology

Two inguinal lymph nodes measuring up to 3 and 4 cm in diameter were removed on August 19, 1976.

Microscopic Findings

The specimen provided for study in this case is from the excisional biopsy of the inguinal mass. The sections revealed diffuse involvement without discernible residual lymph node architecture in most sections. The cellular proliferation is mixed in character with a prominent component of medium size, pale staining cells with abundant cytoplasm. In some of the blocks of this large mass there were residual architectural features in the forms of reactive follicles and intact

121

uninvolved lymph node cortex. In the areas of massive involvement there are numerous small foci of reactive plasma cells, intermixed with the proliferation of cytoplasmic mononuclear cells. The latter cells have nuclei that vary from small to medium size with the nuclei situated somewhat often in a somewhat peripheral or eccentric position. The cytoplasm is pale acidophilic without any evident phagocytosis. The cellular borders at times are fairly sharply demarcated and may present an interlocking pavement-like appearance. Frequently, there are small, irregular lymphocytes intermixed along with cells with elongated fibroblastic-appearing nuclei. There is no distinctive proliferative vascular component. Review of the biopsy of the hilar mass reveals a more prominent fibrillar component with a suggested whirling of cells with elongated fibroblastic type nuclei and an overall appearance suggesting a stromal tumor. The process, however, is also mixed in character and contains the cellular component described in the biopsy of the inguinal mass.

Special Studies

The excisional biopsy of the inguinal mass was performed in an attempt to resolve the diagnostic dilemma. Multiparameter studies revealed that the cells identified as histiocytes definitely stained by alpha naphthyl butyrate for histiocytes. The immunoperoxidase studies for muramidase were prominently positive while those for monospecific immunoglobulin were negative. Immunologic surface marker studies on lymph node suspension revealed a small component of T cells and essentially none of the cells stained with surface immunoglobulin. Ultrastructural studies of this biopsy material failed to reveal any melanosomes within the tumor cells and provided support for the exclusion of the possibility of malignant melanoma. The findings provide support for the histiocyte-monocyte nature of the tumor cells.

The bone biopsy performed at the initial hospital was obtained for review and revealed a diffuse 100% cellularity of the marrow with numerous medium- and large-size cells with abundant cytoplasm. These cells were indistinguishable from the histiocytes found in the lymph node biopsy. The marrow was interpreted as indicating diffuse marrow involvement and provided strong support for the neoplastic nature of this remarkable process.

Histologic Differential Diagnosis

This case presents probably the most difficult differential diagnostic problem in this entire seminar. The histologic problem in the initial hilar lymph node related to the question of whether the process was a malignant neoplasm or a stromal response to a neoplasm because of the unusual mixed cellularity character of the proliferation. The dramatic development of the inguinal mass and the eventual demonstration of a diffuse marrow involvement eliminated the doubt of the neoplastic nature of the process, though the precise classification of the cytologic type was extremely challenging. Three basic processes deserve consideration: (1) an abnormal reaction and inflammation, (2) malignant lymphoma of transformed lymphocytes versus a malignancy of true histiocytic type and (3) a metastatic neoplasm, such as malignant melanoma. A fourth and remote possibility was considered in examining the specimen of the hilar mass, namely, malignant thymoma. Table 1 lists the diagnoses suggested by expert consultation of the lung and mediastinal node biopsy. No definite diagnosis of any of the four diseases was made and all consultants suggested more tissue was necessary for diagnosis.

Considerable difficulty in establishing the diagnosis of malignancy was encountered in both the hilar and inguinal nodes because of the mixed character of the cellular proliferation including histiocytes, lymphocytes, prominent plasma cell component and the lack of pleomorphism of the histiocytic component. On the basis of the histiologic sections of the inguinal mass alone, it is admittedly difficult to establish a diagnosis of malignancy because of the uncertain expressions of

**Table 1. Unusual and Incorrect Diagnosis
Suggested on Lung and Mediastinal Biopsies**

Sclerosing lymphoma
Unusual inflammatory reaction
Metastatic Kaposi sarcoma
Metastatic fibrous histiocytoma

malignant lymphoma of histiocytes at the present time. The lymphoma of transformed lymphocytes, either of large non-cleaved FCC type or immunoblastic sarcoma of T or B cell types, was excluded on the basis of the histiocytic appearance of the medium and large cells. This was later confirmed by the nonspecific esterase and immunoperoxidase studies for muramidase (lysozyme). The third possibility of metastatic melanoma deserves consideration because of the general resemblance of melanoma cells to histiocytes, but the lack of sinusoidal involvement, the intermingling of the apparent tumor cells throughout the node and the cytologic features both on light microscopy and ultrastructural studies exclude malignant melanoma. If the tumor cells were more pleomorphic, cytologic distinction between melanoma and histiocytes might be more difficult. Therefore, special studies for cytologic identification are essential in such situations.

Clinical Staging

The clinically apparent disease both above and below the diaphragm is indicative of clinical stage (CS) III. Biopsy of the hilar and inguinal nodes confirms this and the demonstration of bone marrow involvement establishes this process as pathologic stage (PS) IV. The prominent, initial, febrile symptomatic course of the disease associated with weakness may indicate the B designation, but the possibility of secondary infection must be excluded.

Clinical Correlation and Follow-up

In this case of true histiocytic malignant lymphoma, it is impossible at the present time to consider the clinical correlation because of the rarity of proven cases. Our surface marker studies of 425 cases of non-Hodgkin's lymphomas by 1977 indicates that only one of the 425 cases has been demonstrated to be of true histiocytic type [1]. The present case is the only one found in the 3½-year period. The only point worthy of discussion is how the manifestation in this case compares with the clinical expressions of malignant histiocytosis which is discussed in some detail in the previous case (Case 12). In general, malignant histiocytosis presents with a dramatic onset of a febrile disease commonly associated with hemolytic anemia without masses. This comparison is important, since it appears that malignant histiocytosis may prove to be the most common malignancy of histiocytes, though it, too, is extremely uncommon.

It should be emphasized that it will be some time before a sufficient number of well-documented cases with immunologic surface marker studies and cytochemical procedures are available to define the clinical expressions of true histiocytic lymphoma.

This patient was given chemotherapy (COPP) and recurrence was noted in November 1976. Additional chemotherapy (POMP) was given and only partial response occurred. In December 1976 CVPP and radiation to the scalp and mastoid area were given. In January 1977, huge cervical lymph nodes were noted and ABVD plus prednisone were administered. Dramatic response occurred and in October 1978 (28 months after symptoms) he was doing well with weight gain and hemoglobin of 12.8 gm%. There was no evidence of disease 21 months after the second course of ABVD plus prednisone.

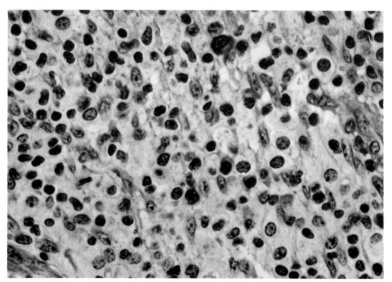

FIG. 1. Malignant lymphoma, histiocytic type: the proliferation is somewhat mixed with prominent clumps of cells, large cytoplasm, round nuclei, and accompanied by fibroblastic cells with elongated oval nuclei and a rare large plasmacytoid cell (H & E 500X).

Reference

1. Lukes, R.J., Parker, J.W., Taylor, C.R. et al: Immunologic approach to non-Hodgkin lymphomas and related leukemias. Analysis of the results of multiparameter studies of 425 cases. Sem. Hematol. 15:322-351, 1978.

Hairy Cell, Leukemia, Spleen

Clinical History

This 69-year-old Caucasian was admitted in February 1975 for elective splenectomy. He had previously a gastroenterostomy for obstructive duodenal ulcer disease. Physical examination indicated the spleen was palpated 4 cm below the right costal margin. Laboratory studies revealed a hemoglobin of 8.8 gm%, hematocrit of 26.6%, MCV of 109 $\mu\mu$g, WBC of 4300 of 91% lymphocytes, 6% neutrophils and 3% monocytes and a platelet count of 137,000/μ^3.

Gross Pathology

A 914 gm multilobular spleen measuring 15.5 × 13.0 × 9.0 cm was removed. The capsule was smooth and red-blue and the cut surface showed rubbery, firm, red-blue tissue.

Microscopic Findings

The initial impression in examining this spleen is that the process is diffuse with the cellular proliferation extending from capsule to capsule. On close inspection, however, with search for Malpighian bodies, these structures are small and almost inapparent and the cellular proliferation is dominantly in the red pulp. The red pulp (particularly with the aid of PAS stain which vividly stains the reticular framework) has a cellular proliferation in the cords of Billroth. Occasionally small clusters of the abnormal cells are found within sinusoids. The cellular proliferation consists of cells with abundant cytoplasm commonly with interlocking cellular borders. The nuclei are oval with fairly uniformly dispersed chromatin and thickened nuclear membranes without prominent nucleoli. The cytoplasm is amorphous and lightly acidophilic and the cellular borders or junctions between cells can be discerned as a fine line. Mitoses are absent. The outstanding feature is the uniformity of the cells and pulp involvement.

Special Studies

The abnormal cells in the *tissue imprints* of the spleen are identical with those found in the peripheral blood and bone marrow. The cells have an amorphous ground-glass appearing pale staining cytoplasm and a round to oval nucleus with finely dispersed chromatin and inapparent nucleoli. At times the nuclei have a deep central indentation passing almost entirely through the nucleus, so that the nucleus appears binucleated or even like a pince-nez. The cytoplasmic border has a variable appearance; it may be finely particulated or have linear or hairy-like extensions, or even be sharply demarcated. It is important to recognize the cells of hairy cell leukemia may be "bald" and not hairy and that other cytoplasmic lymphoid cells may be "hairy." In recent years while reviewing large numbers of cases, it is apparent that the hairiness of the cytoplasmic border is the least reliable criterion for the recognition of hairy cell leukemia. For example, chronic lymphocytic leukemia when cytoplasm is prominent often may have hairy cytoplasmic margins. With the increased recognition of hairy cell leukemia, it has become apparent that most leukemic cells with hairy cytoplasmic borders are not hairy cell leukemias. Therefore, the diagnosis is based upon the cytologic features described and the cytochemical findings.

The presence of tartrate resistant acid phosphatase is essential for establishing the diagnosis of hairy cell leukemia, though admittedly technical problems of fixation or methodology may result in typical cases lacking demonstrable tartrate resistant acid phosphatase. This technique requires the performance of the acid phosphatase procedures twice (once with and the second time without pretreatment with sodium tartrate emersion). Some isoenzymes of acid phosphatase are resistant to prior treatment with sodium tartrate and thus vivid staining occurs in cells containing this isoenzyme. This enzyme may be lost if the cells are not properly fixed or an unduly lengthy period occurs between collection and fixation. This procedure also is effectively utilized on frozen sections of fresh tissue. In the present case the cells in the red pulp stained vividly and even more intensely than those in the peripheral blood. Special studies may be accomplished on air-dried smears or frozen tissue. We have found it possible to mail air-dried smears across the country and still achieve effective results. The non-specific esterase for monocytes is negative. The immuno-peroxidase studies for muramidase or lysozyme are also negative. Thus, there is no support cytochemically for their monocyte nature.

By electron microscopy, low magnification of the hairy cells reveals dramatic numbers of microvilli on their surface. The nuclei are round or oval and have a considerable condensation of chromatin at the nuclear membrane and chromatin aggregations throughout their nuclei. At times deep nuclear clefts are found. The cytoplasm contains varying numbers of mitochondria and in one half of the cases a ribosome-lamellar complex [1]. The cells within the spleen are closely packed and the microvilli are folded and intertwined with the adjacent cells forming an interlocking mesh. This latter feature may account for the "trapping" of the cells within the cords of Billroth. Multiple parameter functional studies were performed on fresh spleen tissue.

Peripheral blood	E	EAC	EA	PV	M	G	A	D	κ	λ
	42	5	0	34	14	35	3	5	31	25
Spleen	19	1	1	74	1	51	3	2	71	32

Over 70% of the cells marked with polyvalent antiserum and 51% marked for the heavy chain IgM, A or D. In the study for light chains 71% marked kappa and 32% lambda. The results indicate the predominant marking as Ig kappa/lambda and suggest the presence of Fc receptor. Of the several cases we have studied, only two or three had marked with monoclonal surface immunoglobulin in support of their B cell nature, while the remainder have marked either in a polyclonal fashion and similar to this case with the Ig kappa/lambda marking. The results in this case do not support the B cell nature of this proliferation. It is possible that the marking with kappa and lambda both is a nonspecific crossover marking, and possibly such cases might be monoclonal IgG kappa. Frozen section with EA rosette technique for monocytes revealed dramatic rosette formation over the areas involved by the hairy cells. This finding would support the histiocyte-monocyte nature of the cells, but the more reliable cytochemical procedure, the alpha naphthyl butyrate, failed to mark the cells as monocytes. There are a small number of cases in the literature, including our own, in which the cells mark in a typical monoclonal fashion [2]. In addition, Dr. Collins from Vanderbilt has been able to strip the immunoglobulin from the surface and demonstrate resynthesis of the monoclonal surface immunoglobulin. Golomb reported resynthesis in all 16 patients tested [2]. This finding provides strong evidence of their B cell origin. However, demonstration of phagocytosis (zymosan particles) in many patients suggests the possible lymphocytes are a special type [2].

Histologic Differential Diagnosis

In the diagnostic evaluation of the spleen consideration is given to whether the process is predominantly in the red or white pulp. The decision whether the process is predominantly red or white pulp is usually easily accomplished, but on occasion is difficult when the white pulp is expanded and includes enlargement of the Malpighian bodies and penicilliary arteriole lymphoid sheaths, so that there may be extensive involvement of the spleen by these areas. Thus, the pathologist needs to identify the splenic arterioles specifically and determine whether the cellularity is above these and extending from these regions into the adjacent tissue or not. Only rarely will the white pulp involvement diffusely involve the spleen without evidence of residual nodularity. In this patient the red pulp is dominantly involved and the white pulp is atrophic. The processes that involve principally the red pulp are granulocytic leukemia, myelomonocytic leukemia, monocytic leukemia and hairy cell leukemia histiocytic medullary reticulosis. The recognition of granulocytic leukemia depends upon finding evidence of granulocytic maturation in the form of myelocytes, metamyelocytes, or eosinophilic myelocytes in the midst of an abnormal mononuclear cell proliferation. The chloroacetate esterase stain is readily accomplished on paraffin sections and is an excellent method for identifying granulopoiesis. Myelomonocytic leukemias also are recognized by their granulocytic features. A true monocytic leukemia of Schilling's type now appears extremely rare and is difficult to recognize with certainty in H & E stained sections. Ideally, it is identified best with cytochemical procedures such as the alpha naphthyl butyrate on touch imprints or frozen sections. In histologic sections the cells appear as large, folded monocytes associated with poorly differentiated mononuclear cells. The diagnosis of histiocytic medullary reticulosis or malignant histiocytosis is described in detail in Case 12. It is based upon three diagnostic features: (1) the recognition of the prohistiocyte, (2) the pleomorphic histiocyte and (3) the mature erythrophagocyte. Chronic lymphocytic leukemia of B cell type and its tissue counterpart malignant lymphoma of the small lymphocytic type also involves the white pulp, but also deserves consideration because the white pulp disease may be extensive and seems to extend into the red pulp. The small lymphocytes, however, are readily distinguishable since they have small- to medium-sized nuclei and scanty cytoplasm without cohesive cellular borders. They generally do not appear to involve the cords of Billroth.

Clinical Staging

Systemic clinical staging in hairy cell disease is never of concern since the disease is initially recognized usually by the finding of the abnormal cells in the peripheral blood and supported by the demonstration of bone marrow involvement. However, "dry tap" is a common experience and if bone biopsy is performed, then marrow involvement is found [2]. Thus, the disease is immediately staged as pathologic stage IV. It is interesting that lymph node biopsies in hairy cell disease are extraordinarily rare. The disease does not present with lymphadenopathy [3]. Even at the time of splenectomy, lymph nodes are rarely removed, apparently since abdominal lymph node enlargement is not encountered.

Clinical Correlation and Follow-up

Hairy cell leukemia is also called leukemic reticuloendotheliosis. The common clinical presentation in hairy cell leukemia is an unexplained prominently enlarged spleen. Often, attention is drawn to the patient because of leukopenia, anemia or pancytopenia. Search of the peripheral smear will often reveal the typical hairy cells. The tartrate resistant acid phosphatase procedure is extremely important in this situation to provide absolute confirmation of the cytologic identity, particularly if the pathologist is not well acquainted with the cytologic features. At times the cells may present in leukemia proportions with rare cases over $100,000/mm^3$. With prominent splenomegaly and peripheral blood involvement, the marrow essentially is always involved [3]. It is readily demonstrated in Jamshidi needle biopsies or marrow particle sections as cohesive aggregates of mononuclear cells with abundant cytoplasm similar to those found in the spleen. Usually little or no hematopoiesis is found because of the extensive marrow involvement. We have encountered cases in which the uninvolved portions of the marrow are hypoplastic.

It is more than three years after splenectomy, and the patient is doing well with hemoglobin of 16.7 gm%, WBC of 9000 cells/mm^3 and platelets of $240,000/mm^3$.

Summary

The basic nature of this process is unknown, though it presently appears to involve a special B lymphocyte. Whether this process properly belongs within the leukemias can be debated. This is emphasized by the realization recently that a number of cases improve after splenectomy and seem to be nonprogressive; whereas, the disease manifestations may rapidly deteriorate with chemotherapy. It is puzzling that in this process that bears a leukemic designation we are still uncertain what is the normal counterpart cell. We have not observed any association with other disorders of the B cell system. Furthermore, the peripheral blood involvement by the abnormal cell is usual but in moderate to low numbers. Thus, the status of hairy cell leukemia is unsettled.

References

1. Golomb, H.M. and Vardiman, J.: Hairy cell leukemia: Diagnosis and management. CA 28:265-277, 1978.
2. Golomb, H.M.: Hairy cell leukemia: An unusual lymphoproliferative disease. A study of 24 patients. Cancer 42:946-956, 1978.
3. Katayama, I. and Finkel, H.E.: Leukemic reticuloendotheliosis. A clinicopathologic study with review of the literature. Am. J. Med. 57:115-126, 1974.

V
Abnormal Immune Reactions: Imitators of Hodgkin's Disease

Introduction

Hodgkin's disease is one of the remarkable disorders of medicine, not only because of its varied clinical disease expressions, but also because of its diversity of morphologic features. As a result of this diversity of expression, Hodgkin's disease causes major problems in differential diagnosis, since it may be simulated by a wide variety of disorders from benign immune reactions at one extreme to a variety of types of malignant tumors. The principal reason for the diagnostic difficulty is that lobated nuclei, binucleated, multinucleated and pleomorphic cells resembling diagnostic Reed-Sternberg cells may be found under a variety of conditions of both benign reactive processes and malignant neoplasms of diverse type. Our recent proposal is accepted that Reed-Sternberg cells are not pathognomonic of Hodgkin's disease [1]. Furthermore, the diagnosis of Hodgkin's disease is no longer based only on the finding of Reed-Sternberg cells, but the occurrence of diagnostic Reed-Sternberg cells with large nucleoli in association with the morphologic findings of one of the histologic subtypes.

In Table 1, the histologic expressions of Hodgkin's disease are grouped by histologic types and the lesions which may most commonly simulate specific histologic types. The general morphologic features that raise the possibility of Hodgkin's disease can be considered by histologic pattern and include (1) mixed cellularity, (2) prominent proliferation of lymphocytes with or without histiocytes, (3) lesions containing large cells some of which exhibit lobation, binucleation or multinucleation and (4) prominent fibrosis. From a perusal of this table, it is apparent that almost any lymph node proliferation that alters the architecture focally, partially or extensively may resemble Hodgkin's disease. In severe reactive processes of lymphoid tissue, the interfollicular tissue may contain exaggerated foci of immunoblastic reaction containing large transformed lymphocytes with nuclear lobation or multinucleated large cells, and in this manner resemble focal partial involvement of the lymph

135

Table 1. Imitators of Hodgkin's Disease

Prominent Histologic Features	Hodgkin's Expressions	Subtype of Hodgkin's Disease	Imitators of Hodgkin's Disease
Mixed cellularity nodular	Paracortical T cell zone, focal or partial involvement	Mixed	Reactive hyperplasia
	Nodular	Nodular sclerosis	FCC lymphomas
Mixed cell: "histiocytic"	Predominately lymphocytic proliferation with or without histiocytes	L & H	Lennert group
	Sarcoid histiocyte clusters, histiocyte aggregates	L & H	Toxoplasmosis
	Histiocytes – eosinophils fibrosis in varying	Mixed	Allergic granulomatosis

	Lacunar cell	Nodular sclerosis	Infectious mono.
			Abnormal immune reaction
	Pleomorphic	Lymphocyte depletion (Reticular)	IBL-like disorders hypersensitivity IBS variety of large malignant histiocytes
Fibrosis	Capsular sclerosis	Nodular sclerosis	Sclerosing inflammatory lesions
	Disorderly fibrosis throughout node (poorly formed)	Lymphocyte depletion (Diffuse fibrosis)	Metastatic lympho-epithelioma with sclerosis and eosinophils

L&H = Lymphocytic and histiocytic types of Hodgkin's disease.
FCC = Follicular center cell lymphomas.
IB = Immunoblasts.
IBL = Immunoblastic lymphadenopathy.
IBS = Immunoblastic sarcoma.

node. Sometimes Hodgkin's disease initially involves the node in the paracortical or T cell zone. Lymphomas of follicular center cell type, particularly with a large cleaved FCC component, may have large and irregular or even polypoid cells that at times closely resemble Reed-Sternberg cells. Commonly, these large cells are situated within the center of lymphomatous follicles and thus present a nodular proliferation that may be mistaken for the vaguely nodular pattern of L & H (lymphocyte predominance) Hodgkin's disease. Another group where lymphocytes and histiocytes are prominent in varying proportions produces the so-called Lennert's lesion and has caused great difficulty in recent years, since its description [2]. These will be described in detail in case 22. This "Lennert lesion" demonstrates a problem of differential diagnosis because Professor Lennert apparently included five lesions within the group and now it is apparent that one is Hodgkin's disease. Toxoplasmosis may present problems because of the prominent histiocytic component expanding the interfollicular tissue. Usually it can be readily recognized because of the prominent reactive follicular hyperplasia associated with clusters of histiocytes in the lymphocytic mantle and in intrafollicular locations. In the histologic group with mixtures of cells, a problem arises if prominent fibrosis, reactive histiocytes and eosinophilia are present. Allergic granulomatosis, eosinophilic granuloma of lymph nodes and a variety of reactions associated with hypersensitivity are considered in the differential diagnosis of such a combination. The lymph node of allergic granulomatosis contains distinctive "allergic" granulomas, while eosinophilic granuloma is primarily a sinusoidal histiocyte reaction associated with eosinophils. Hodgkin's disease, by contrast, essentially does not involve lymph node sinusoids. Hodgkin's disease seems to spare sinusoids for a reason that is unknown, and if "Reed-Sternberg cells" are found within sinusoids, a primary consideration should be given to a malignant histiocytosis. In another group which has prominent large cells with nuclear lobation and multinucleation, the list of lesions simulating Hodgkin's disease is long. They include both normal reactions such as post vaccination lymphadenitis, infectious mononucleosis, Herpes zoster, and the abnormal immune reactions (including immunoblastic lymphadenopathy in a wide variety of associated abnormal immune reactions); immunoblastic sarcoma, malignant histiocytosis, and a variety of tumors involving lymph nodes in which the tumor cells have prominent lobated nuclei, multinucleation, or produce Reed-Sternberg-like cells. Obviously, the differential diagnosis is extremely difficult at times and depends upon a thorough understanding and appreciation of the criteria for each of the histologic types of Hodgkin's disease. In the sclerosing group, a wide variety of lesions may be encountered, both benign and malignant type, in which fibrosis is prominent. Sclerosing inflammatory lesions, particularly if eosinophils, are prominent, present considerable difficulty for the pathologist, since any process of this type will often have numerous immunoblasts with prominent nucleoli. An unusual but important lesion of this group is the metastatic nasopharyngeal carcinoma (lymphoepithelioma) that may be associated with dramatic sclerosis and eosinophilia. This process may cause particular difficulty, since the epithelial component may represent the least prominent component or be limited to only portions of the tumor.

It was impossible to include representative samples of all groups of the imitators of Hodgkin's disease for this seminar, and three unusual examples were selected to illustrate the range of lesions that may resemble Hodgkin's disease.

References

1. Lukes, R.J., Tindle, B.H. and Parker, J.W.: Reed-Sternberg-like cells in infectious mononucleosis. Lancet 2:1003, 1965.
2. Lennert, K. and Mestdagh, J.: Lymphogranulomatosen mit konstant hohem Epitheloidzellgehalt. Virch. Arch. Abt. A. Path. Anat. 344:1-20, 1968.

Abnormal Immune Reaction (With Histiocytic Component), Axillary Lymph Node

Clinical History

This 72-year-old male had been in generally good health except for recent episodes of easy fatigability. In the previous two to three months, he also experienced diaphoretic episodes of 24 to 28 hours duration. Inguinal lymphadenopathy had been noted during the previous 15 years. In January 1974 he underwent a tonsillectomy for enlarged tonsils and recurrent tonsillitis. Six months later in July, a lymph node from the right neck region was biopsied and interpreted as atypical lymphoid hyperplasia.

The current biopsy material ,was obtained February 19, 1976. Physical examination revealed a 2 cm nodule over the left parotid gland, a 4 X 3 cm tender nodule in the left axilla and a 3 X 2 cm nodule in the left groin. There was no splenomegaly but the liver was palpated three fingerbreadths below the right costal margin. A biopsy of the axilla and left groin was performed.

Gross Pathology

The specimen was several circumscribed nodules of soft homogenous, yellow stained pink fragments, measuring up to 6 X 4 X 3 cm. The cut surface revealed several areas of hemorrhage measuring up to 7 mm in greatest dimension.

Microscopic Findings

The biopsy reveals a mixed cellular proliferation without discernible lymph node architectural features. There is extension of the lymphoid tissue into the adjacent adipose tissue. Throughout the specimen there is a variable component of

141

histiocytes aggregated for the most part in small cohesive clusters. These clusters usually are aggregates of two to eight cells in diameter and rarely exceed a high magnification field in size. The small clusters of histiocytes are separated by lymphocytes in which an occasional vessel is discernible but few large cells are obvious. On higher magnification the histiocytes have abundant acidophilic cytoplasm, round to oval nucleoli and finely dispersed chromatin and often a small central sharply demarcated nucleolus. Occasionally, the histiocytes contain nuclear debris in their cytoplasm, but essentially the cytoplasm is devoid of phagocytic material. The proliferation between the histiocyte clusters is composed predominately of lymphocytes that have round regular nuclei and fairly compact basophilic chromatin without apparent nucleoli. Eosinophils are occasionally scattered throughout the infiltrate in small numbers, and larger cells with features of immunoblasts are found. None of the cells resemble the Reed-Sternberg cell variants. Plasma cells are occasionally noted.

In summary, the lesion consists of a prominent component of reactive epithelioid histiocytes arranged in small clusters in association with a small round lymphocyte component with small numbers of immunoblasts, plasma cells, eosinophils, but without any cells that resemble Reed-Sternberg cells or Reed-Sternberg cell variants.

Special Studies

Cell suspensions were obtained from the lymph node biopsies for immunologic surface marker studies at the Sutter Community Hospital (Frank Glassy, M.D.) and performed by Dr. M. R. MacKenzie at the University of California, Davis. The results reveal the findings similar to those that we have observed in the study of 68 cases with reactive lymph nodes. Forty-one percent of the cells marked as B cells in a polyclonal fashion and 52% as T cells with E rosettes. We did not, however, have the opportunity to study the lymphocytes either in imprints, cytochemical methods or in cytocentrifuge preparations.

Histologic Differential Diagnosis

The diagnosis in cases of this type is difficult since there are a variety of lesions that are associated with a reactive histiocyte component and specifically with epithelioid clusters. The differential diagnosis is listed in Table 1. The frequency of histiocytes and their aggregations admittedly varies in all the lesions; therefore, it is dangerous to rely strongly on the character of the histiocyte aggregation. It is essential to base the differential diagnosis on the proliferation accompanying the histiocytes. Lennert's lesion is an example of this problem in which the original report was based upon the epithelioid aggregates rather than distinguishing the processes based on the accompanying cellular proliferation. Thus the Lennert lesion as a result has caused considerable problems in understanding the process and in the differential diagnosis. The lesion reported by Lennert appears to include Hodgkin's disease of lymphocytic and histiocytic type, abnormal immune reactions with reactive histiocyte component, toxoplasmosis and IBL when histiocytes are prominent and a specific type of T cell lymphoma that usually has an epithelioid histiocyte component. The recognition of these lesions is dependent upon having fairly ideally collected and processed histologic material. Unfortunately, much of the consultation material we receive from pathologists around the

Table 1. Histologic Categories of the "Lennert Lesion"

Hodgkin's L & H Type	L & H variant of Reed-Sternberg cells
	Diagnostic Reed-Sternberg cells
	Nodular lymphocyte proliferation
Toxoplasmosis	Follicular hyperplasia
	Histiocyte clusters, intra and perifollicular
Abnormal immune reactions	Diffusely involved node
	IB and plasma cells
IBL with histiocytes	(1) arborizing PAS + thick walled vascular proliferation
	(2) IB and plasma cells
	(3) Deposit of amorphous acidophilic inter. material
ML, T cell type with epithelioid histiocytes	Medium-sized lymphocytes with irregular twisted nuclei
	Occasional immunoblasts

IBL = Immunoblastic lymphadenopathy.
IB = Immunoblast.

country is considerably less than optimum, and this histologic differentiation is extremely difficult even when the essential criteria for differentiation are well known to the observer. There are also several other lesions that deserve consideration and include the so-called nonspecific granulomas described initially in laparotomy specimens, spleen, abdominal lymph nodes and liver in patients with Hodgkin's disease; familial histiocytosis; and the noncaseating granulomas. In this presentation we will primarily be concerned with those processes included in the Lennert's lesion as pointed out by Tindle and Long [1].

Clinical Staging

Not applicable in benign process.

Clinical Correlation and Follow-up

In the interim since the publication of the Lennert lesion (1968) it has become increasingly apparent that the group was heterogeneous. At the present time we and others are attempting to determine the significance of the groups included within the Lennert lesion, i.e., those processes associated with epithelioid clusters. The significance of lymphocytic and histiocytic Hodgkin's disease is now well known. The cases with proven toxoplasmosis are not a problem, but those lymphomas which have serologic evidence of active toxoplasmosis are a different problem. Because of the immunosuppressive character of chemotherapy agents and the immunologic vulnerability of patients with lymphomas, toxoplasmosis should be treated initially and the lymphoma subsequently to prevent dissemination of toxoplasmosis. There is a broad group of abnormal immune reactions that we are just becoming acquainted with and learning to recognize. Immunoblastic lymphadenopathy appears to be a rather distinctive entity within this group and possibly the extreme type of proliferation that is usually progressive. At the present time approximately 10% of these have progressed to immunoblastic sarcoma in our large series. The abnormal immune reactions may represent a variety of disorders some of which may be related to IBL as less severe and reversible expressions. Undoubtedly it will be some time before sufficient numbers of cases have been evaluated in depth with newer immunologic techniques before this entire group is defined. Finally, the new T cell lymphoma associated with histiocytes that we have studied appear to be the distinctive lymphoma group within the Lennert lesion. The four cases included within our report have not fared well clinically, two having progressed rapidly to immunoblastic sarcoma, the third having died within the year following multiple agent chemotherapy. The process is generalized when initially observed at biopsy, but possibly may have had a prolonged initial phase as an abnormal immune reaction. With this small number of cases evaluated thus far it is impossible to define the clinical expressions.

The patient was doing well as of March 1978.

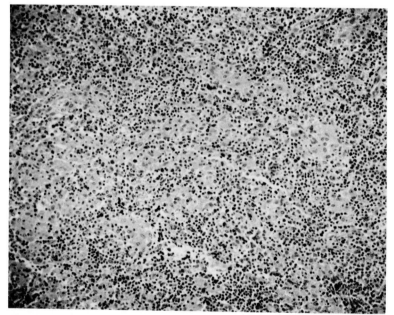

FIG. 1. Abnormal immune reaction: the cellular proliferation presents a Lennert-like appearance with prominent clusters of epithelioid histiocytes of varying size separated by predominantly lymphocytic proliferation (H & E 50×).

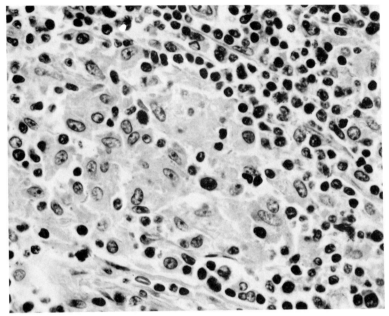

FIG. 2. Between and around the histiocyte clusters are lymphocytes and immunoblasts and a few eosinophils (H & E 500×).

Reference

1. Tindle, B.H. and Long, J.C.: CPC. 30-1977. N. Engl. J. Med. 297:206-211, 1977.

Abnormal Immune Reaction, Immunoblastic (Immunoblastic Lymphadenopathy-like), Cervical Lymph Node

Clinical History

This 30-year-old black female was admitted in August 1976 for fever, diarrhea, painful lymphadenopathy and rash which began on the back and spread over the entire body. Nausea and vomiting with right upper quadrant pain had been present for three to four months. She had a two-year history of blackout spells and one resulted in an auto accident. A neurologist had placed her on Dilantin therapy for blackout spells. Physical examination revealed a generalized maculopapular rash involving the trunk, face and extremities. There was generalized tender lymphadenopathy involving cervical axillary and inguinal nodes. Laboratory data revealed a hemoglobin of 13.8 gm% and WBC of 29,400. The differential count was 24 PMNs, 10 bands, 56 lymphocytes, 1 eosinophil and 9 monos. A right cervical lymph node was removed.

Gross Pathology

The specimen was several cervical nodes measuring 2.5 × 1.5 × 1.0 cm.

Microscopic Findings

The specimen consists of a lymph node with discernible peripheral sinuses but essentially without any reactive follicles. There is a definite increase in number of small vessels that is much more apparent in PAS stained sections. The vessel walls are slightly to moderately thickened by a deposit of PAS positive material and the endothelium is at times hyper-

147

plastic. The cellular proliferation is mixed in character and consists of small irregular lymphocytes and medium to large immunoblasts. These cells had finely distributed nuclear chromatin, frequently two prominent nucleoli on the nuclear membrane and abundant amphophilic cytoplasm. In methyl green pyronine stains the immunoblasts are dramatically demonstrated and are numerous in areas. Sinusoids frequently contain numerous immunoblasts along with many small lymphocytes. Plasma cells are irregularly dispersed throughout the infiltrate and are most common in the medullary portions. There are numerous interspersed reactive histiocytes with pale staining cytoplasm and oval to folded monocytoid nuclei that impart the multiple pale staining foci to the cellular infiltrate. The cellular proliferation is diffuse in character for the most part and either compresses the sinusoids or the sinusoids are filled with cells and rather inapparent. Mitoses are numerous. There is no amorphous pale staining interstitial material. There are no cells resembling Reed-Sternberg cells.

Special Studies

Examination of the peripheral blood at the time of the lymph node biopsy revealed circulating numerous plasmacytoid lymphocytes. Functional studies of the lymph node revealed only a small number of B cells (6%), a normal number of T cells (72%) and over 20% unmarked cells. The unmarked cells may be plasma cells. The low number of marked B cells may relate to the infrequency of reactive follicles noted histologically. There were too few cells for a complete study.

Lymph node	E	EAC	EA	PV	M	G	A	D	κ	λ
	72	20	2	6	ND	ND	ND	ND	ND	ND

Histologic Differential Diagnosis

This diffusely involved lymph node with the prominent immunoblastic component and a somewhat prominent vascular proliferation of small vessels raises the possibility of immunoblastic lymphadenopathy and Hodgkin's disease. Of secondary concern with any immunoblastic proliferation is infectious mononucleosis and vaccination lymphadenopathy. With the prominent histiocyte component, toxoplasmosis also deserves consideration. In toxoplasmosis there is a prominent component of follicular hyperplasia and the histiocytes are characteristically situated in clusters in the lymphocytic mantle and in the follicular center, though they may be found also in the interfollicular areas. Infectious mononucleosis usually has a follicular component but it dramatically involves the interfollicular tissue by a marked immunoblastic proliferation with intermediate forms between the small lymphocyte and the immunoblast and component. This proliferation reflects in our view the varying stages in lymphocyte transformation from the small lymphocyte to the fully transformed cell. Associated with this evidence of B cell transformation towards plasma cell is the cytoplasmic lymphocyte of the Downey type with prominent pale staining cytoplasm and small- to medium-sized lymphocyte nuclei. The cells are often intermingled with the immunoblasts, but also are found in the lymph node sinuses. In post vaccination lymphadenitis the process is dominantly small lymphocytes and immunoblasts with the immunoblasts at times involving almost entire portions of the nodes and in this way resembles a monoclonal proliferation or neoplasm. The cytologic features of the immunoblasts, however, are normal in appearance. The two processes of major concern are more difficult to exclude. In Hodgkin's disease we encounter large abnormal mononuclear cells that resemble to some degree immunoblasts and Reed-Sternberg cell variants which we have interpreted as polypoid transformed lymphocytes (immunoblasts). These include the L & H variant and lacunar cells and the diagnostic Reed-Sternberg cell. Because large immunoblasts may have prominent nucleoli and in severe immunoblastic reaction they may be multinucleated and even be accompanied by cells that fulfill the criteria for diagnostic Reed-Sternberg cells, this differentiation may be extremely difficult, particularly if the material is not collected and processed optimally. In our opinion the Reed-Sternberg cells of infectious mononucleosis have nucleoli with tinctorial qualities that are indistinguishable from those in Hodgkin's disease and cannot be validly distinguished by staining procedures. Thus, the distinction between Hodgkin's disease and immunoblastic proliferations with diagnostic Reed-Sternberg cells is based on the associated cellular proliferation. For example, are there Reed-Sternberg cell variants and the features of the Hodgkin's process or are there features of less abnormal immunoblastic proliferation, such as infectious mononucleosis? This distinction represents one of the most challenging diagnostic problems in lymph node pathology and requires considerable experience. In considering the possibility of immunoblastic lymphadenopathy (IBL), this case clearly does not fulfill the three criteria we described: (1) the diffuse involvement of the node by a striking arborizing vascular proliferation; (2) the dramatic immunoblastic and plasma cell proliferation; and (3) the deposit of acidophilic interstitial material that is associated with a generally hypocellular lymph node. In this case there is no deposit of interstitial amorphous material and the immunoblastic proliferation though prominent is not as severe in IBL. Furthermore, there is a lack of arborizing vascular proliferation. It is acknowledged that the process may represent a mild form of immunoblastic lymphadenopathy that may subside upon withdrawal of Dilantin or with mild therapy only to be retriggered at some later date by Dilantin or some other sensitizing agent, at which time the characteristic degree of these changes might be evident. The morphologic features in cases such as this strongly suggest that minor degrees of IBL exist and are likely to go unrecognized. We have chosen to regard this degree of lymph node change as abnormal immune reaction and that the morphologic findings are only reliable when observed in severe degrees. In addition, these features of IBL appear to represent a hypersensitive lymphadenopathy process that may be encountered with a variety of agents.

Clinical Correlation and Follow-up

The Dilantin therapy was stopped and the rash disappeared. The lymphadenopathy regressed and she did well. Subsequently she had rash, fever and chills with lymphadenopathy which also regressed. As of October 1977 she was alive and well. The immunologic stimulation noted in this lymph node may be related to the possible drug abuse suspected in this patient. Caution must be given, since some examples of Dilantin lymphadenopathy may have progressed to lymphoma according to some reports although we have not seen such examples.

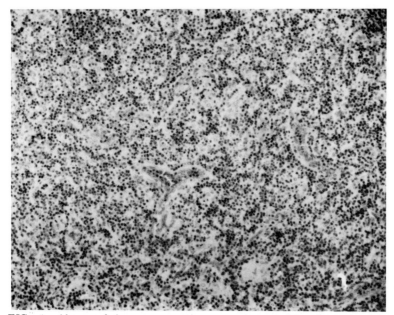

FIG. 1. Abnormal immune reaction: process consists of a mixed infiltrate with a prominent vascular component and hyperplastic endothelial cells (H & E 50×).

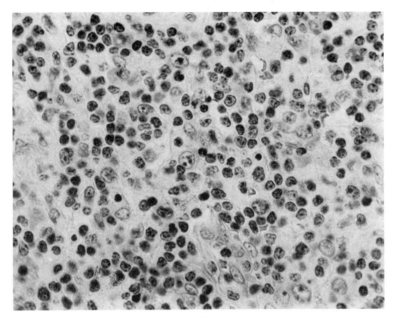

FIG. 2. Number of immunoblasts with round oval nuclei, finely dispersed chromatin and one or several nucleoli present. Cytoplasm is basophilic and ill-defined. Small lymphocytes vary somewhat in nuclear configuration (H & E 500×).

Bibliography

Hyman, G.A. and Sommers, S.C.: The development of Hodgkin's disease and lymphoma during anticonvulsant therapy. Blood 28:416-427, 1966.

Lukes, R.J. and Tindle, B.: Immunoblastic lymphadenopathy: A hyperimmune entity resembling Hodgkin's disease. N. Engl. J. Med. 292:1-8, 1975.

Saltzstein, S.L. and Ackerman, L.V.: Lymphadenopathy induced by anticonvulsant drugs and mimicking clinically and pathologically malignant lymphomas. Cancer 12:164-182, 1959.

Metastatic Carcinoma (Lymphoepithelioma) With Sclerosis and Eosinophilia, Neck Mass

Clinical History

This 14-year-old black male was well until two months prior to admission when he developed flu. A mass appeared on the left side of his neck after a few days. Following ampicillin treatment, no improvement was noted and the mass increased in size. In April 1976 a cervical lymph node showed reactive hyperplasia. He also complained of anorexia, epistaxis, decrease in hearing and dysphasia. Physical examination revealed an 8 × 7 × 4 cm mass which was palpated over the right sternocleido-mastoid muscle extending 2 cm above the right clavicle. Several shotty right supraclavicular and inguinal lymph nodes were palpated. A tumor was excised from the right neck along with several cervical lymph nodes.

Gross Pathology

The specimen was a mass measuring 4 × 6 cm which had a tan nodular surface. There were multiple fibrous bands and areas of necrosis within the mass.

Microscopic Findings

This process consists of a markedly variable mass without discernible lymph node architecture in which there are varying degrees of sclerosis and at times remarkable degrees of tissue eosinophils. The sclerosis varies from advanced degrees almost devoid of cellularity to fibrillary connective tissue that contains a mixed cellular infiltrate. Eosinophilia is prominent throughout, but in areas there are almost pools of eosinophils and at times associated with peculiar necrosis that stains in a distinctive amphophilic manner. The remaining cellular proliferation varies also extensively and contains variable numbers of large mononuclear cells with prominent nucleoli; at times these occur in clusters that on close inspection appear to be a cytoplasmic syncytium about which eosinophils often are dramatic in numbers. The cytoplasm is amphophilic and finely granular and the cytoplasmic borders are ill-defined in some areas. Occasionally, the syncytial areas have two nuclei that are closely situated and the cells may appear binucleated and closely resemble diagnostic Reed-Sternberg cells with huge nucleoli. The variability in the appearance of this process caused us considerable difficulty in diagnosis. Over 40 histologic blocks were prepared and examined, and in a limited number of these there were small cystic structures lined by large cells resembling those in the syncytium previously mentioned. In a few areas the syncytial aggregates of cells had almost a serpentine arrangement with well-defined margins. Small reactive follicles were present in some areas. The initial lymph node biopsy revealed features of reactive hyperplasia with secondary reaction centers. The lymph node capsule was dramatically altered. These findings suggest that the initial lymph node was situated in the periphery of the mass and only the capsular portion was involved. Upon close inspection of the lining of the cyst, the cells are clearly arranged in an epithelial arrangement and there is a suggestion of polarity though cellular borders are usually not well defined and the epithelium has a syncytial appearance. This small area is the diagnostic clue for metastatic squamous carcinoma.

Special Studies

Immunologic surface marker studies were performed on a lymph node and portion of the neck mass. In both specimens there was difficulty obtaining sufficient numbers of cells for a complete evaluation. In both specimens there was a large number of unmarked cells and in the lymph node a marked reduction in the number of cells forming E rosettes, while in the lymph node a number of cells with surface immunoglobulin for T cells were within the normal range.

Lymph node	E	EAC	EA	PV	M	G	A	D	κ	λ
	17	6	0	29	ND	ND	ND	ND	ND	ND
Neck mass	32	20	0	ND	ND	ND	ND	ND	ND	ND

Histologic Differential Diagnosis

There are four principal areas of concern in the differential diagnosis as follows: (1) Hodgkin's disease — the histologic types of Hodgkin's disease, particularly nodular sclerosis; (2) abnormal immune reactions, specifically immunoblastic lymphadenopathy and including hypersensitivity phenomenon to therapeutic agents; (3) the response to parasitic infestations, such as filariasis; and (4) metastatic lymphoepithelioma. This case, because of the dramatic degrees of sclerosis and eosinophilia, is easily confused with Hodgkin's disease of nodular sclerosing type. The wide areas of sclerosis and even sclerosing bands necessitate consideration of Hodgkin's disease. The isolated large mononuclear cells and cells closely mimicking Reed-Sternberg cells obviously make this distinction difficult. Of additional concern was the small amount of epithelial components. In this case, the epithelial component was found in approximately six of the 40 blocks and inapparent in the majority. The typical serpentine arrangement of the metastatic nasopharyngeal carcinoma (lymphoepithelioma) was limited to a single block in this case. In nodular sclerosis the cohesive clusters of lacunar cells present an epithelial-like appearance to an individual with limited experience and often concern for a metastatic carcinoma with sclerosis is acknowledged. The critical differentiation in this case depends upon identifying syncytial epithelium or, if fortunate, the epithelial lining of a cystic space, whereas Hodgkin's disease is based upon critical use of the criteria for lacunar cells. Abnormal immune reactions, particularly with clinically evident hypersensitivity, may have dramatic eosinophilia and varying degrees of fibrosis. Usually in this situation, lymph node architecture is still discernible and the typical triad of immunoblastic lymphadenopathy is present to some degree. Vascular proliferation involving small arborizing vessels and the varying degrees of immunoblastic proliferation are usually found. In this case, immunoblastic proliferation is present, but vascular proliferation was not impressive. The amorphous acidophilic material is also lacking. The third possibility, a reaction to a parasite, always deserves consideration whenever tissue eosinophilia is dramatic. Filariasis produces the most dramatic degree of eosinophilia of any known parasite and is commonly associated with marked degrees of sclerosis of the capsule. In the tissue surrounding lymph node an adult parasite may be found. Eosinophilia may occur in remarkable degrees in a node and the microfilarial forms may even produce eosinophilic abscesses. Manifestations of other parasites in lymph nodes are extremely uncommon. Usually, no parasite is found even though the general character of the process suggests a parasitic etiology. Another process producing severe eosinophilia and fibrosis with resultant mass formation is the so-called allergic granulomatosis of Churg and Strauss in which the lymph node architecture may be totally altered. The process is readily identified by the presence of allergic granulomas. These structures are small and have characteristic amphophilic staining amorphous central material with a narrow zone of marginating epithelioid cells. Earlier stages of this may reveal partially necrotic eosinophils centrally. Allergic granulomas of lymph nodes deserve consideration only because of the intense eosinophilia and necrosis. This process in our experience can readily be differentiated since it is essentially a severe proliferation of the littoral cells of the sinusoids associated with central necrosis and an intense eosinophilia. Sclerosis is usually absent. The necrotic areas within the sinusoids may involve degenerating eosinophils and lend an amphophilic character to the amorphous necrotic material. The finding of poorly differentiated squamous carcinoma in one block provides the accurate diagnosis although the clinical proof of a primary site was lacking.

Clinical Staging

Staging laparotomy was performed and spleen and lymph nodes showed no evidence of metastatic tumor.

Clinical Correlation and Follow-up

Biopsy of the nasopharynx was refused by the parents because the child was very frightened and anxious. Radiation therapy was given to the nasopharyngeal area. Subsequently, a nose bleed occurred and blind biopsies of the turbinates were performed. These small tissues revealed poorly differentiated squamous carcinoma and this area was not included in the irradiated area. After consultation, a surgical resection of the lateral nasal wall with removal of the inferior and medial turbinates was performed. Chemotherapy had been initiated but, with the documented biopsy proof of primary squamous carcinoma, chemotherapy was stopped (May 1977). Subsequently, in June, left neck enlargement was noted and in August 1977, a modified neck dissection was done. Five of 38 lymph nodes contained metastatic poorly differentiated squamous carcinoma. In the fall, right neck mass became palpable and chemotherapy was started again because it seemd that once chemotherapy was stopped (May 1977), the tumor became more apparent. However, the patient had an allergic reaction and chemotherapy was given cautiously. The right neck mass enlarged and radiation was given. As of October 1978, there is no clinical evidence of tumor.

The clinical presentation in this case is unusual. A large mass apparently in the midneck at the region of the sternocleidomastoid muscle is quite different from the usual single large node near the angle of the mandible where nasopharyngeal carcinoma usually causes lymph node enlargement. Through the years, however, we have had the opportunity to study approximately ten cases of metastatic lymphoepithelioma with sclerosis and eosinophilia and they have all been in children. In one, the lesion was situated in the midline of the suboccipital region which is the lymphatic drainage from the nasal pharynx. In the others, the precise location is uncertain, but was in the general upper cervical region.

The huge size of this mass suggests that it may well have occupied the majority of the cervical region on that side. Unfortunately, the nasopharynx and tonsillar regions were only visually inspected and the clinicians were reluctant to perform a random biopsy because of the hyperactive state of the patient at the time of the inspection. In cases of this type, a random biopsy is critical since the process in our experience has often been multicentric and superficial and the direct visualization has failed to reveal any obvious evidence of tumor.

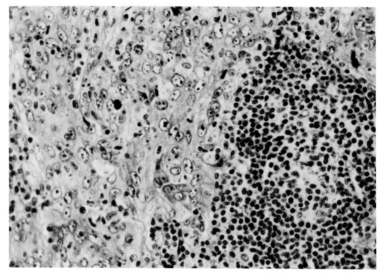

FIG. 1. Metastatic carcinoma: tumor is composed predominantly of syncytial epithelial cells with round to oval nuclei with highly dispersed chromatin and one or several small nucleoli. Small amount of residual lymphoid tissue remains (H & E 125×).

VI
Hodgkin's Disease

Introduction: Historical Notes

The unique combined inflammatory and neoplastic-like features of Hodgkin's disease have fascinated generations of clinicians and pathologists in the almost 150 years since Thomas Hodgkin published his original paper in 1832 entitled, "Some Morbid Appearances of the *Absorbent* Glands and Spleen" [1]. The investigation of Hodgkin's disease in the century and a half can be divided into four eras: (1) the early clinical and pathologic descriptions, (2) the search for an etiologic agent, (3) the recognition of the immune defect and (4) the beginning of the modern era of clinical and pathologic description and effective therapy. Thomas Hodgkin is recognized for his original appreciation of the distinctness of the disease separating the involvement of lymph nodes and spleen from inflammation. The importance of this observation was emphasized by Wilks who extended and confirmed the Hodgkin's observation and gave the disease its eponymic designation. The initial microscopic descriptions in surprising detail were initially provided by Greenfield, who appreciated not only the mixed character of the proliferation but described eosinophils, giant cells and fibrosis [2]. To close out the era of the initial clinical and pathologic descriptions it is well known that Sternberg and Reed described the cytologic features of the diagnostic cell which bears their names. It is generally unappreciated that they held conflicting views of the etiology of the process with Sternberg being convinced of the tuberculous nature of the process, while Reed held a remarkable appreciation of its immunologic alteration, though not in modern terminology [3]. In the second era, the search for an etiologic agent, exhaustive attempts were made to find an etiologic agent. In the early portion of this period, there were staunch supporters such as Sternberg for its tuberculous etiology. Later investigators were convinced of its relationship to brucellosis, and for decades the belief persisted that the etiology was an atypical mycobacterium. In the third period, the recognition of an immune defect began with the observation

161

of anergy in patients with Hodgkin's disease by Parker, Jackson and associates in 1932 [4]. Cutaneous reactivity to antigens was found to be diminished in Hodgkin's disease [5]. The demonstration of the loss of delayed hypersensitivity responsiveness in experiments of homograft rejection was published in 1958 by Kelly et al [6]. Thus there is abundant evidence that there is an immunologic defect in Hodgkin's disease, but whether this defect is primary or secondary is not resolved.

The beginning of the modern era of clinical and pathologic description of Hodgkin's disease began with the work of Jackson and Parker who rekindled interest in this disorder [7]. They defined the morphologic features of three histologic types — paragranuloma, granuloma and sarcoma — and demonstrated the evolution of the process from the early or so-called benign form, paragranuloma, to the classical granuloma, to the rapidly fatal sarcoma and related them to their clinical manifestations.

The modern era of therapy began with a Swiss radiologist, Rene Gilbert, who demonstrated the improved effectiveness of intense radiation therapy and also the orderly proximal spread of the disease. From these observations, Peters developed the systematic assessment of the disease as clinical staging and demonstrated the effectiveness of radiation therapy for treating the involved area and proximal fields [8]. The histologic types of Hodgkin's disease described by Lukes and Butler which redefined the pathology of Hodgkin's disease related the pathologic manifestations to the clinical stage of the disease and survival [9]. These advances in Hodgkin's disease, together with the proposal of its potential curability, led to the Rye Conference and a redefinition of clinical stages and a systematic approach to the evaluation of Hodgkin's disease. The six histologic types of Lukes and Butler were condensed to four types at the Rye Conference for ease of clinical application [10]. Following the Rye Conference, the widespread use of lymphangiography revealed the retroperitoneal involvement in Hodgkin's disease that was undetectable by previous techniques. The recognition of the pattern of sequential spread accounts for the development of exploratory laparotomy as a means of determining involvement precisely of retroperitoneal lymph nodes, spleen, liver and bone marrow. With these laparotomy results, previously undetected areas of abdominal involvement have been included in irradiation therapy fields and a significant improvement in the effectiveness of therapy occurred. In the Ann Arbor Conference of 1971, the definition of clinical staging recognized that localized extralymphatic involvement did not alter the clinical stage. Separation of those cases staged by clinical and exploratory laparotomy was designated as clinical stage and pathological stage. This means of detecting precisely the extent of disease has been paralleled by the improvement in radiation therapy and combination chemotherapy.

Median survival of Hodgkin's disease of all types has been reported in excess of 80%.and disease-free survival beyond 60%. Unfortunately, this improved effectiveness has been achieved not without a high price of second malignancies and more recently by the observation of myeloblastic leukemias occurring in patients treated wtih combined radiation therapy and chemotherapy [12]. With the exception of this single blemish, the successful redefinition of the clinical and pathologic manifestations of Hodgkin's disease, a systematic evaluation of the disease by teams of clinical investigators and the dramatic improvement of therapy have been an unparalleled success story in the field of cancer.

HISTORICAL ASPECTS OF HODGKIN'S DISEASE

I. *Initial Clinical and Pathologic Descriptions*

   1832 Thomas Hodgkin's initial description
   1865 confirmation and named
   1878 Greenfield; initial microscopic description
   1889 Sternberg)
   1902 Reed   )description of characteristic giant cell

II. *Search for an Etiologic Agent*

   1880 present: exhaustive search

III. *Recognition of Immune Defect*

   1931 Jackson & Parker
   1956 Schier et al; Delayed Hypersensitivity
   1958 Kelly et al; Homograft Rejection

IV. *Modern Era of Clinical and Pathologic Description and Therapy*

1937-1944 Jackson & Parker; Clinical Pathologic Description
1950 Peters; Staging & Systematic Radiation Therapy
1960s Kaplan; Megalovoltage Therapy of Hodgkin's Disease
1966 Lukes and Butler; New Classification
1970s Ann Arbor; Staging Refined

References

1. Ober, W.B.: Hodgkin's disease. Historical notes. New York State J. Med. 77:126-133, 1977.
2. Greenfield, W.S.: Specimens illustrative of the pathology of lymphadenoma and leucocythaemia. Trans. Path. Soc. London 29:272-304, 1878.
3. Reed, D.M.: On The Pathological Changes in Hodgkin's Disease with Especial Reference to its Relation to Tuberculosis. Johns Hopkins Hospital Report 10:133-196, 1902.
4. Parker, F., Jr., Jackson, H., Jr., Fitz Hugh, G. et al: Studies of disease of the lymphoid and myeloid tissues. IV. Skin reactions to human and avian tuberculin. J. Immunol. 277-282, 1932.
5. Schier, W.W., Roth, A., Ostroff, G. et al: Hodgkin's disease and immunity. Am. J. Med. 20:94-99, 1956.
6. Kelly, W.D., Lamb, D.L., Varco, R.L. et al: An investigation of Hodgkin's disease with respect to the problem of homotransplantation. Ann. N.Y. Acad. Sci. 87:187-202, 1960.
7. Jackson, H., Jr., and Parker, F., Jr.: Hodgkin's disease. I. General consideration. N. Engl. J. Med. 230:1-8, 1944.
8. Peters, M.V.: Study of survivals in Hodgkin's disease treated radiologically. Am. J. Roentgenol. 63:299, 1950.
9. Lukes, R.J. and Butler, J.J.: The pathology and nomenclature of Hodgkin's disease. Cancer Res. 26:1063, 1966.
10. Lukes, R.J. et al: Report of the Nomenclature Committee. Cancer Res. 26:1311, 1966.
11. Lukes, R.J.: Criteria for involvement of lymph node, bone marrow, spleen and liver in Hodgkin's disease. Cancer Res. 31:1755-1767, 1971.
12. Coleman, C.N., Williams, C.J., Flint, A. et al: Hematologic neoplasia in patients treated for Hodgkin's disease. N. Engl. J. Med. 297:1249-1252, 1977.

Hodgkin's Disease, Lymphocyte Predominance (Lymphocytic and Histiocytic, Nodular), Axillary Lymph Node

Clinical History

A 15-year-old black female had an axillary lymph node biopsy in 1968 following a dog bite. Histologic interpretation was benign reactive hyperplasia. In September 1975 an axillary lump was excised which had been present for "several years." Several 1.5 to 2.0 cm firm, movable, nontender masses were palpated in the right axilla. Chest radiograph was normal and laboratory data included a hemoglobin of 12.8 gm%, WBC 7400 with a differential of 39 PMNs, 58 lymphocytes, 2 monocytes and 1 eosinophil.

Gross Pathology

A soft yellow-tan 3.0 × 2.5 × 2.5 cm lymph node was removed which contained thin fibrous bands that separated small nodules within the node.

Microscopic Findings

The lymph node architecture is considerably distorted by a nodular proliferation that extends irregularly throughout the node. Several small unaltered reactive follicles may be noted in the compressed peripheral portion of the node. The large ill-defined nodules that lack a lymphocytic mantle are occasionally vaguely outlined and may be difficult to discern. The nodules are composed of a variable mixture of lymphocytes and histiocytes. The histiocytes occur singly or in small clusters. Within the nodules are varying numbers of large mononuclear cells with lobated nuclei and a limited amount of pale cytoplasm. These have been termed the L & H variant of the Reed-Sternberg cell and have finely dispersed chromatin, multilobated overlapping twisted nuclei and small or inapparent nuclei. Occasional cells contain a prominent nucleolus, and a rare mononuclear cell will show a large or huge nucleolus. Careful search of multiple sections fails to reveal classical diagnostic Reed-Sternberg cells with the mirror-image nuclei and huge nucleoli. Therefore, in this patient with the general features of Hodgkin's disease, typical diagnostic cells were not noted. An occasional area in the node shows a slight increase in perivascular connective tissue but no definite areas of fibrosis. Focal necrosis is absent. The capsule is intact and the medullary sinuses are not apparent. The vessels are not prominent. Methyl green pyronine (MGP) sections show that the mononuclear cells with prominent nucleoli have pyroninophilic cytoplasm of limited amount, whereas the L & H variants have no or a minimal amount of pyroninophilia. Lymphocytes throughout the proliferation are small, irregular and occasionally have peculiar configurations. The chromatin is finely dispersed and a small dotlike nucleolus is often present. These lymphocyte features are in contrast to the typical small round lymphocyte that have compact nuclear chromatin and inapparent nucleoli. The diagnostic criteria for the histologic diagnosis are listed in Table 1.

Table 1. Lymphocyte Predominance (L & H Nodular)[1]

Architecture	Obliterated
Follicles	Few in residual compressed node
Nodules	Large, vaguely outlined
Cellularity	Lymphocytes and histiocytes in varying proportions
	Eosinophils few
Fibrosis	Typically absent
Necrosis	None
R-S Cells	Diagnostic type rare
	L& H variant numerous

Special Studies

Immunologic surface marker studies on the axillary lymph node and porta hepatis lymph nodes and the uninvolved portions of the spleen are shown below:

	E	EAC	EA	PV	M	G	A	D	κ	λ
Lymph node	85	40	8	6	4	5	0	6	3	5
Lymph node	91	26	21	1	1	0	0	2	1	0
Spleen (A)	88	19	16	11	9	3	0	7	10	4
Spleen (B)	85	14	0	15	11	5	0	7	10	5

The marker studies in the four specimens are similar. There is a
high percentage of E rosettes in each specimen and few cells
with surface immunoglobulin. These findings indicate a predominant T cell component and indicate that the lymphocyte
response in Hodgkin's disease is predominately a T cell type. It
is interesting in that there is a disproportionate number of cells
forming EAC (complement dependent) rosettes in relation to
those positive with polyvalent antiserum for B lymphocytes.
This observation suggests that T lymphocytes in lymph nodes
may possess a complement receptor. These cells have been
considered prethymic T lymphocytes and we as well as others
have noted the complement receptor on the convoluted T cell
lymphoma cells also.

Staging

Twenty-one days following the axillary node biopsy, an exploratory staging laparotomy was performed. The spleen
weighed 220 gm and contained multiple pale nodules varying
from 0.2 to 2.0 cm. Microscopically, the nodules were composed of small lymphocytes, similar to the lymph nodes along
with scattered L & H variants of the Reed-Sternberg cells and
several diagnostic Reed-Sternberg cells. The splenic hilar and
portal hepatis lymph nodes were similarly involved but not
impressively enlarged. The celiac, periaortic, right and left iliac
and mesenteric nodes exhibited features of reactive hyperplasia.
The portal areas of the liver in both the needle and wedge liver
biopsies contain lymphocytic infiltrates without any Reed-
Sternberg cells or related mononuclear forms. The bone marrow
was normal. This finding indicates clinical stage IA but pathological stage III$_S$.

Clinical Correlation and Follow-up

Patients with lymphocyte predominance most commonly present as young males under 30 years of age. The cervical region usually is noted to contain single large nodes, high in the neck adjacent to salivary glands. Clinical staging frequently indicates the disease is most commonly stage I and therapy presents the best chance for prolonged survival and even cure. In this case, a young female with axillary lymph node presentation has an unusual extent of disease with both abdominal lymph nodes and spleen involvement. The prognostic significance of these widely separate involved structures in lymphocyte predominance type of Hodgkin's disease is presently not known. The prognosis for prolonged therapy as performed in this case may be suggested by the recent data from the Stanford University Medical Center. An 89% five-year survival for all histologic types of Hodgkin's disease was found when combined chemotherapy and radiation therapy was applied. However, it is too early to evaluate ten-year survivals and potential cure rates in the favorable histologic types.

This patient was treated with combination chemotherapy (COPP) followed by radiation therapy to both the upper mantle and an inverted Y. At three years she was doing well without evidence of disease (November 1978).

Reference

1. Lukes, R.J.: Criteria for involvement of lymph node, bone marrow, spleen, and liver in Hodgkin's disease. Cancer Res. 31:1755-1767, 1971.

FIG. 1. Hodgkin's disease — L & H type: vaguely outlined nodule in L & H
Hodgkin's disease is composed of a mixture of small lymphocytes and pale
cytoplasmic reactive histiocytes with a few large intermixed forms of cells
(H & E 12.5×).

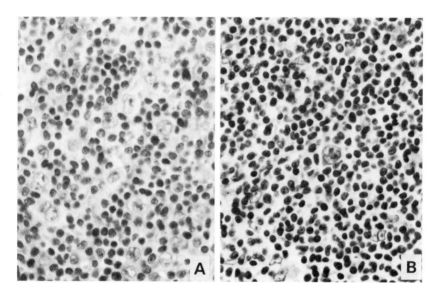

FIG. 2. (A) Intermixed L & H variants of Reed-Sternberg cells have large
irregular to multilobated or overlapping nuclei with finely dispersed
chromatin and small nucleoli. The cytoplasm is pale and fairly abundant
(H & E 500×). (B) A bilobated form with prominent nuclei is suggestive of
a diagnostic Reed-Sternberg cell (H & E 500×).

Hodgkin's Disease, Lymphocyte Predominance (Lymphocytic and Histiocytic, Diffuse, Aggressive), Cervical Lymph Node

Clinical History

A 53-year-old male noted a cystic mass in the left neck region three years prior to excision which was considered to be a brachial cleft cyst. Aspiration revealed no fluid. There was no other cervical or generalized lymphadenopathy. The excised nodal material measured up to 4.5 cm in greatest dimension and included fragments with an irregular nodular surface. Laboratory studies were normal including a hemoglobin, WBC, although the ESR was 46 mm/hr.

Microscopic Findings

The large lymph nodes have a broadly thickened capsule, and are diffusely involved by a mixed cellular proliferation without any suggestion of nodularity. The cellular proliferation is composed of lymphocytes and large reactive histiocytes and variable numbers of large cells are intermingled, some of which are multinucleated. The large cells predominately have pale staining chromatin, small nucleoli and often twisted and overlapping the nuclei with a small amount of pale staining acidophilic cytoplasm. The cytoplasm at times is vacuolated at the periphery, bringing to mind lacunar cells, but there is no well-defined acidophilic cell membrane at the margin. With lymphocytes adjacent to this large cell, the space appears to be artifactual. In some sections these large cells have acidophilic to amphophilic cytoplasm and prominent nucleoli. The number of such cells are variable in multiple sections. The cytoplasm and nucleoli of these cells are prominently pyroninophilic in contrast to those with pale staining cytoplasm. The prominence of these large nucleolated cells suggests an aggressive type of lymphocytic and histiocytic Hodgkin's disease which is more likely to have involvement beyond the region of presentation with extension to the abdomen and spleen. The histiocytes have abundant, pale, acidophilic cytoplasm, and large oval nuclei with finely dispersed nuclear chromatin and small nucleoli. These cells often occur in cohesive groups and even epithelioid-appearing clusters. The lymphocytes are small and irregular and at times have a peculiar twisted configuration. Plasma cells are infrequent and there is little or no fibrosis. Necrosis is absent. Pertinent morphologic criteria are listed below in Table 1.

Special Studies

None performed.

Staging

At exploratory laparotomy, the lymph nodes of the abdomen were small and difficult to find and microscopically proved to be uninvolved. The spleen weighed 192 gm and microscopically lacked any evidence of Hodgkin's disease. The needle and wedge biopsies of the liver and bone marrow did not reveal any evidence of involvement. These results indicate CS IA and PS IA.

Table 1. Lymphocyte Predominance (L & H, Diffuse)*

Architecture	Obliterated
Follicles	Few or absent
Nodules	Usually none
Cellularity	Lymphocytes and histiocytes in varying proportions
	Eosinophils few, occasionally numerous
Fibrosis	Typically absent
Necrosis	None
R-S Cells	Diagnostic type typically rare; increased frequency indicates mixed type
	L & H variant numerous

*Lukes, R.J.: Criteria for involvement of lymph node, bone marrow, spleen and liver in Hodgkin's disease. *Cancer Res.* 31:1755-1767, 1971.

Clinical Correlation and Follow-up

Several months following laparotomy, the patient completed "spade" radiation of 4000 rads. Later progressively enlarged left cervical and inguinal adenopathy was palpated. In subsequent months there was waxing and waning of the node size and eventually the nodes became small and not palpable. The patient was seen approximately a year following laparotomy, in good health and ESR of 19 mm/hr. There were two episodes of pericarditis, possibly related to radiation. The serum copper remained in the normal range. At 3½ years, there was no evidence of recurrent disease.

The clinical setting for lymphocyte predominance — Hodgkin's disease with diffuse node involvement — is similar to that of the nodular subtype although the nodular subtype usually indicates a more prolonged survival. Also, the nodular subtype may have a higher incidence of clinical stage I than the diffuse, and the disease may be less aggressive. However, there are no large series available and at the present time no information regarding differences in therapy has been published.

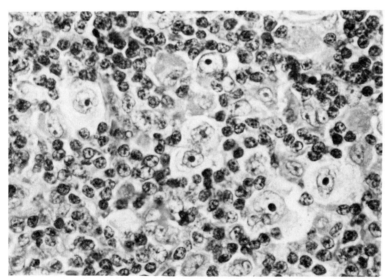

FIG. 1. Hodgkin's disease — L & H type: numerous large cytoplasmic cells that are lobated or binucleated with prominent nucleoli are found within a lymphocytic proliferation (H & E 500×).

Hodgkin's Disease, Mixed, Cervical Lymph Node

Clinical History

A 5½-year-old Puerto Rican girl noted an enlarging mass in the right neck for three months. No recent immunizations were known. There was no fever, night sweats, anorexia or weight loss. Physical examination revealed an 8 × 4 cm smooth mass in the right neck. Cervical lymph nodes, a few epitrochear lymph nodes and inguinal lymph nodes were also palpated although the liver and spleen were not palpated. Laboratory studies were within normal limits except for an ESR of 32 mm/hr. The chest radiograph showed a questionable right mediastinal shadow.

Gross Pathology

A gray, soft lymph node measuring 5.5 × 2.5 × 2.0 cm was removed from the right neck.

Microscopic Findings

The lymph node is partially involved by a variable cellular proliferation that extends through the interfollicular and paracortical region surrounding and isolating reactive follicles with their surrounding lymphocytic mantles. The cellularity varies from area to area with prominance of histiocytes in areas and of lymphocytes in other areas. Scattered throughout the infiltrate are prominent large cells and variable numbers of eosinophils. The large cells are both mononuclear and polypoid and a number have prominent or even huge nucleoli, the latter being associated with amphophilic cytoplasm. Diagnostic Reed-Sternberg cells with abundant amphophilic cytoplasm and multilobated nuclei with huge nucleoli are readily found. The morphologic critiera are summarized in Table 1.

Table 1. Mixed Cellularity

Architecture	Diffusely obliterated
Cellularity	Partial involvement common
	Varies widely; may resemble L & H diffuse fibrosis, and reticular types
R-S Cells	Diagnostic type frequent or numerous
	Includes unclassifiable lesions.

Special Studies

Immunologic surface marker studies were not performed because this specimen was from a distant area (New York). Immunoperoxidase studies for cytoplasmic immunoglobulin using monospecific antikappa and antilambda antisera revealed that the diagnostic Reed-Sternberg cells contain both kappa and lambda light chains similar to that reported by Anagnostou et al [1].

Staging

Exploratory laparotomy for staging was performed and no evidence of abdominal disease was noted. This indicates clinical stage IA and pathologic stage IA.

Clinical Correlation and Follow-up

No follow-up information is available. Childhood Hodgkin's disease through the decades has generally been regarded to have a poor prognosis and is associated with progressive disease and ineffective therapy. Recently, it has been emphasized that there is a distinctive difference between Hodgkin's disease in children below the age of 10 years or prior to puberty as compared with those older than 10 or postpubertal. The latter have the general histologic features and type of disease resembling adult Hodgkin's disease. In addition, there is considerable difference in the frequency of Hodgkin's disease in the first decade when compared to the decade beyond. The histologic presentation in childhood has recently been reviewed by Rappaport, Strum [2] and by Butler [3]. These studies reveal male predominance and nodular sclerosis and lymphocyte predominance subtypes. A poor prognosis is expected if the patient is below 10 years of age or has clinical stage II or III disease. Because of the deleterious effect of radiation therapy on growth, development, function, oncogenesis, genetic consequences, multiple agent chemotherapy, accurate staging of childhood Hodgkin's disease is especially important. Approximately 40% of children subjected to laparotomy in clinical stages I, II and III had a different pathological stage [4]. Reed-Sternberg cells and lacunar cells have been noted to contain cytoplasmic immunoglobulin and this supports the hypothesis that Reed-Sternberg cells are transformed B lymphocytes. However, the apparent presence of kappa and lambda light chains has been difficult to explain unless the cytoplasmic immunoglobulin is bitypic, i.e., a single light chain with antigenic determinants for both kappa and lambda light chains. Opponents of this view base their objections on the possibility that the immunoglobulin is not synthesized by the Reed-Sternberg cells, but is the result of pinocytosis. Others adhere to the view that the Reed-Sternberg cell is a neoplastic polypoid histiocyte. A recent study of in vitro immunoglobulin synthesis by Reed-Sternberg cells supports the macrophage derivation hypothesis [5].

Therapy of childhood Hodgkin's disease has previously been reported with dismal results. For example, the five-year survival in one series of 44 patients reported in 1959 was 18%. However, in a recent study reported by Rosenberg, the five-year actuarial survival was 89% [6]. In their series of 79 patients, 41 had laparotomy and 31% had a change in stage following the laparotomy. In order to maximize the quality of survival, low dose radiation and MOPP chemotherapy was proposed. A different chemotherapeutic regimen has been evaluated at Memorial Sloan-Kettering Cancer Center [7]. Results of involved field radiation therapy for early stage Hodgkin's disease has been evaluated [8]. New regimes of therapy are also under consideration such as radiation therapy as the initial therapy and chemotherapy for relapse. Long-term follow-up is important because a second malignant tumor may occur. In the series of 116 children reported from Mayo Clinic, 29 survived beyond ten years and three of these patients developed another malignant tumor (acute myelomonocytic leukemia, carcinoma of the breast, and thyroid carcinoma) [9].

References

1. Anagnostou, D., Parker, J.W., Taylor, C.R. and Lukes, R.J.: Lacunar cells of nodular sclerosing Hodgkin's disease. An ultrastructural and immunohistologic study. Cancer 39:1032-1043, 1977.
2. Strum, S.B. and Rappaport, H.: Hodgkin's disease in the first decade of life. Ped. 46:748-759, 1971.
3. Butler, J.J.: Hodgkin's disease in children. *In* Neoplasia in Childhood. Chicago:Year Book Medical Publishers, 1969.
4. Hays, D.M.: The staging of Hodgkin's disease in children reviewed. Cancer 35:973-978, 1975.
5. Kadin, M.E., Stites, D.P., Levy, R. et al: Exogenous immunoglobulin and the macrophage origin of Reed-Sternberg cells in Hodgkin's disease. N. Engl. J. Med. 299:1208-1214, 1978.
6. Donaldson, S.S., Glatstein, E. and Rosenberg, S.A.: Pediatric Hodgkin's disease. II. Results of therapy. Cancer 37:2436-2447, 1976.
7. Tan, C., D'Angio, G.J. and Exelby, P.R.: The changing management of childhood Hodgkin's disease. Cancer 35:808-816, 1975.
8. Cham, W.C., Tan, C.T.C., Martinez, A. et al: Involved field radiation therapy for early stage Hodgkin's disease in children. Preliminary results. Cancer 37:1625-1632, 1976.
9. Norris, D.G., Burgert, Jr., E.O., Cooper, H.A. et al: Hodgkin's disease in childhood. Cancer 36:2109-2120, 1975.

Hodgkin's Disease, Lymphocyte Depletion (Reticular), Supraclavicular Lymph Node

Clinical History

A 36-year-old female experienced weight loss and fever for three months. She had right upper quadrant pain for two years. A brother, stepsister and stepmother's daughter died of Hodgkin's disease. She was hospitalized for diagnostic tests but refused lymph node biopsy on several occasions. Laboratory data included a hemoglobin of 3.3 gm%, WBC of 7100 cells/mm^3. The differential count was 88 PMNs, 6 bands, 5 lymphocytes, 6 monocytes. The absolute lymphocyte count was 355 cells/mm^3. The reticulocyte count was 11.3% and the anemia was interpreted as normochromic, normocytic. A cervical lymph node measuring 4.5 × 2.8 × 1.8 cm was removed and the tissue was pale gray-tan. The chest radiograph indicated pleural effusion and mediastinal mass that may have been adenopathy. A liver-spleen scan revealed hepatosplenomegaly with impaired hepatic function. A biopsy was performed on March 24, 1976.

Gross Pathology

The largest lymph nodes measured 4.5 × 2.8 × 1.8 cm and all were pale tan.

Microscopic Findings

The specimen consists of an infiltrative mass without discernible architectural features indicative of lymph node. Extending through the mass is a variable cellular proliferation including a dramatic component in many areas of large abnormal mononuclear cells, and large cells with multilobation and multinucleation with prominent nucleoli. A number of the

179

mononuclear cells have two or three small nucleoli and resemble immunoblasts. The lobated and multinucleated cells have densely amphophilic cytoplasm and the MGP stains showed the mononuclear and multinucleated cells are strikingly amphophilic. Many of the mononuclear cells and multinucleated cells contain large to even huge inclusion-like nucleoli. Plasma cells are numerous in some foci. The process has varied expressions and many large cells are interpreted as Reed-Sternberg cell variants and diagnostic Reed-Sternberg cells with huge nuclei. Lymphocytes are infrequent and connective tissue is limited to the perivascular hyalinized type. The morphologic criteria are recorded in Table 1.

Table 1. Lymphocyte Depletion (Reticular) [1]

Observed in 2 forms:	
1. Predominance of diagnostic R-S cells	
2. Sarcomatous R-S cells predominate	
Architecture	Partially to totally obliterated
Cellularity	Depends on type
	Disorderly nonbirefringent
Fibrosis	Prominent if lesion overlaps with diffuse fibrosis type

Special Studies

The immunologic surface marker studies were difficult to accomplish because of the abundance of cellular debris and the results require special interpretation. Sheep erythrocyte rosettes for T cells were performed and revealed 86% of cells formed rosettes. However, the variable number of residual cells for study in the cytocentrifuge preparation were principally small lymphocyte type. The remaining rosette studies and procedures for determining surface immunoglobulins were not positive, possibly because of the rapid tumor cell death. The immunoperoxidase studies for cytoplasmic immunoglobulin revealed that the large multinucleated cells believed to be Reed-Sternberg cells contained both kappa and lambda chains which we have found typical of these cells. Thus the surface marker studies reflect the T cell response and do not characterize the tumor cells.

Lymph node	E	EAC	EA	PV	M	G	A	D	κ	λ
	86	*	*	*	*	*	*	*	*	*

Histologic Differential Diagnosis

This case is considered to fulfill the criteria for the reticular type of Hodgkin's disease since the predominant proliferative cell exhibits expressions of the diagnostic Reed-Sternberg cell with amphophilic and pyroninophilic cytoplasm and huge nucleoli. The histologic differential diagnosis in such cases may be extremely difficult and includes the pleomorphic expressions of both B and T cell lymphomas, including the immunoblastic sarcoma, large noncleaved follicular center cell and the pleomorphic expressions of a number of malignant tumors including carcinoma and sarcoma. The infiltrative aggressive form of nodular sclerosis subtype of Hodgkin's disease also must be considered. In both the lymphomas and non-lymphomatous tumors, a precise diagnosis must depend upon finding areas of more recognizable, less pleomorphic tumor or evidence in previous biopsies of more typical diagnostic expressions of these specific neoplasms. In this case the diagnosis is based upon varied expressions of the Reed-Sternberg cells which predominate throughout the proliferation. Of great interest in this case is the finding of cytoplasmic immunoglobulin which we believe is characteristic of the Reed-Sternberg cell [2].

Staging

A random Jamshedi needle biopsy of the marrow revealed extensive necrosis and involvement by a similar cellular proliferation. Therefore, this patient had clinical stage and pathological stage IVB.

Clinical Correlation and Follow-up

The follow-up in this patient indicates the patient died nine months following diagnosis and an autopsy was not performed. Lymphocyte depletion Hodgkin's disease appears to be a distinctive entity from our recent study [3]. The patients are

---

*Impossible because of cellular debris.

primarily older males with a median age of 57 years and they usually present with an abdominal mass. There is usually little or no peripheral lymphadenopathy. The histologic expression in ten of the 13 cases was a diffuse fibrosis and the remaining three cases exhibited the reticular type. The disease at autopsy was limited to the abdomen, abdominal lymph nodes, spleen, liver and bone marrow. The laboratory findings revealed there was a consistent lymphocytopenia as well as pancytopenia in almost every case before therapy. Thus, in lymphocyte depletion, not only is there a loss of circulating lymphocytes, but damage to the hematopoietic system with frequent severe marrow hypoplasia before therapy. The disease is rapidly progressive with a median survival of four months, and in every patient death occurred within nine months. The present case has a number of atypical features that caused us to reexamine the diagnostic possibilities. This patient was a female below the age of 40 who presented with a mediastinal mass and supraclavicular lymph nodes. This is atypical for lymphocyte depletion type and is more characteristic of nodular sclerosis. With this clinical presentation, an aggressive pleomorphic type of nodular sclerosis must be considered. The host response may be ineffective and the typical lacunar cells and sclerosing may also reflect ineffective host response and the histologic pattern and clinical setting of aggressive type of nodular sclerosis may be indistinguishable from lymphocyte depletion Hodgkin's disease. We have coded this as lymphocyte depletion but recognize that exclusion of a nodular sclerosis variant is difficult.

References

1. Lukes, R.J.: Criteria for involvement of lymph node, bone marrow, spleen, and liver in Hodgkin's disease. Cancer Res. 31:1755-1767, 1971.
2. Anagnostou, D., Parker, J.W., Taylor, C.R. et al: Lacunar cells of nodular sclerosing Hodgkin's disease. An ultrastructural and immunohistologic study. Cancer 39:1032-1043, 1977.
3. Neiman, R.S., Rosen, P.J., and Lukes, R.J.: Lymphocyte-depletion Hodgkin's disease. A clinicopathologic entity. N. Engl. J. Med. 288:751-755, 1973.